Dealing with Life Challenges:

Fatigue Management, Stress, and Mental Health

Joseph Leutzinger, Ph.D.

Kane Miller, M.S.

Tracy Sladek, B.S.

*Special thanks to Dr. Dennis W. Holland, Union Pacific Railroad
for his editorial and scientific review assistance*

Published by

Table of Contents

Chapter 1 - What is Fatigue?

Fatigue is a condition, or state-of-being, that every adult has experienced in their lifetime. It often occurs in response to physical exertion, lack of sleep, or high emotional stress level and can also be associated with other health problems. Weakness, drowsiness, and fatigue are terms often used interchangeably. However, weakness and drowsiness are actually symptoms associated with fatigue. A universally accepted definition for fatigue is weariness from bodily or mental exertion.

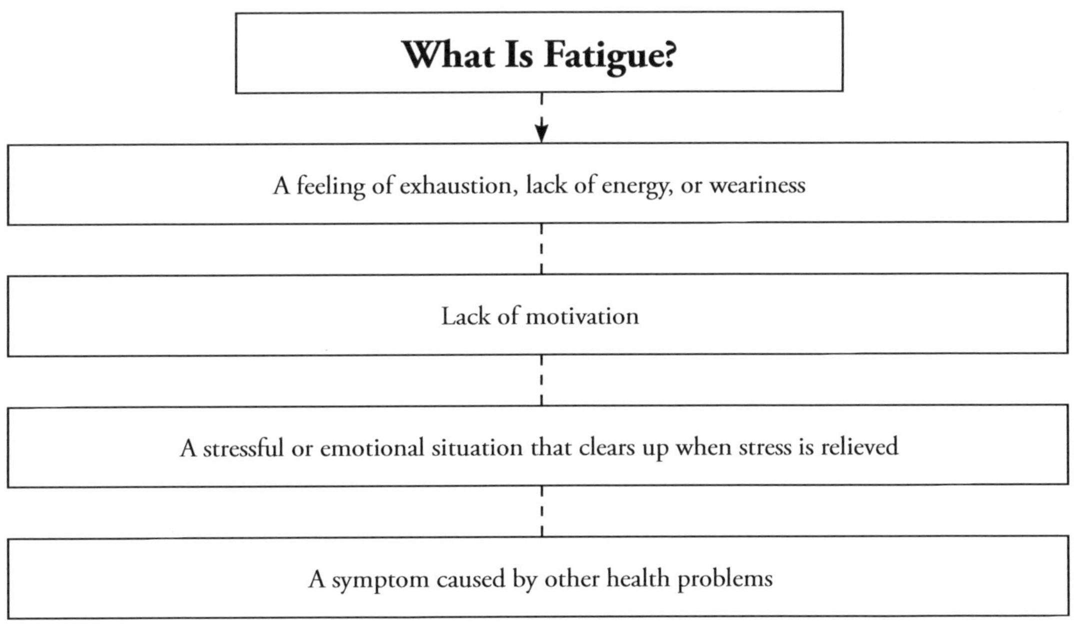

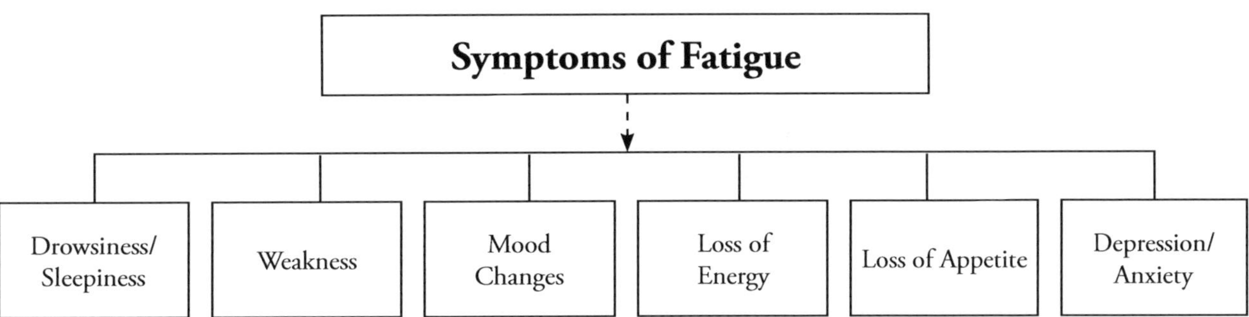

Fatigue is one way your body may communicate to you that something is wrong when physical and mental abnormalities occur, making fatigue a vital part of life. Fatigue can become problematic if ignored, or when it is not relieved by sleep, stress management techniques, or other health improvement behaviors. Fatigue affects people in different ways. Mood changes, loss of energy, loss of appetite, inability to focus, and difficulty remembering are some of the many potential symptoms or conditions that may result from fatigue.

There are several possible physical and psychological causes of fatigue such as anemia, persistent pain, sleep disorders, regular use of alcohol or drugs, diabetes, cancer, arthritis, and other diseases. Another common source of fatigue is a disruption of an individual's internal clock or circadian rhythm – a daily rhythmic activity cycle, based on 24-hour intervals.

It takes about 20 days for the circadian rhythm to adjust if the same sleep schedule is followed over that time. However, shift workers may have varied or erratic schedules so it may not be possible to maintain the same sleep schedules. Fortunately there are guidelines available that can help to reduce or prevent fatigue among shift workers.

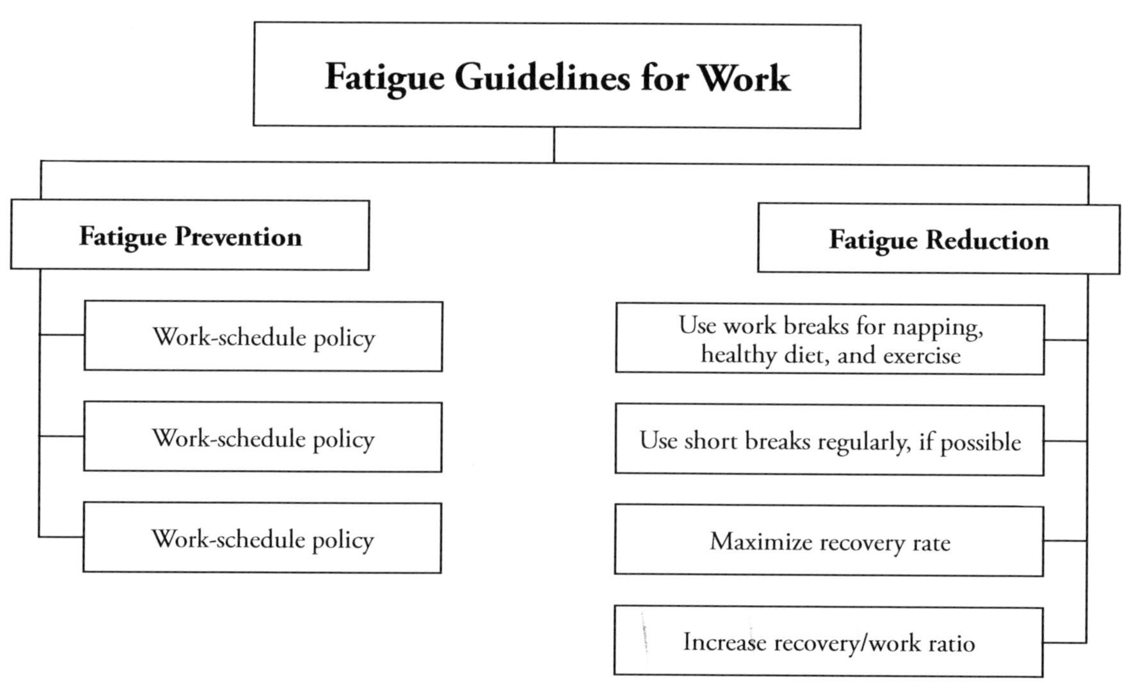

Insomnia

Fatigue is a primary symptom of insomnia and other sleep disorders, such as sleep apnea, restless leg syndrome, and disruption of the circadian rhythm. The "Issues Surrounding Fatigue" schematic provides an overview of sleep disorders and insomnia.

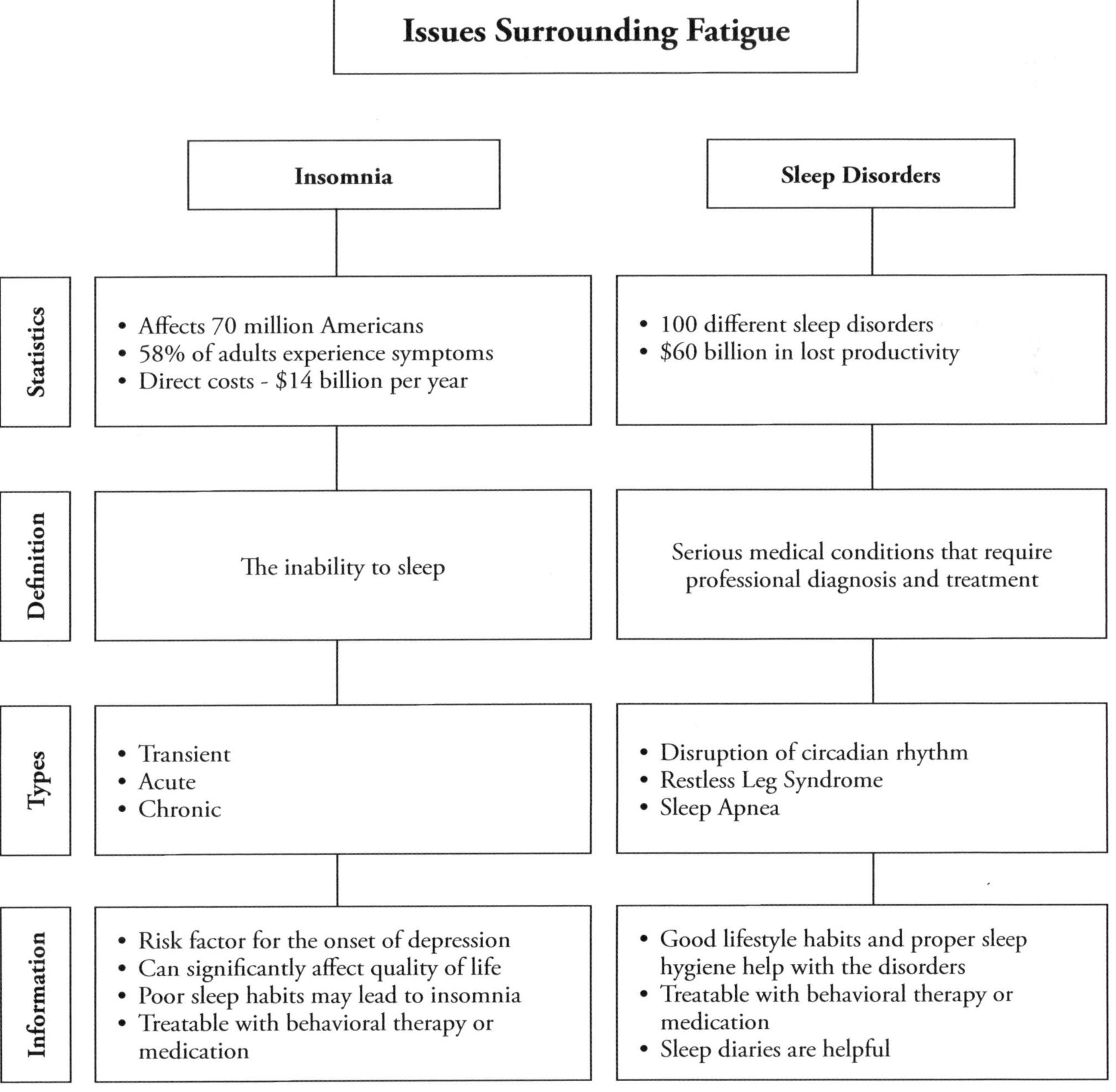

Over 70 million Americans are affected by insomnia, according to the National Institutes of Health. Currently $14 billion is spent annually on the direct costs of insomnia (i.e. treatment, health care services, hospital care, and nursing home care). Insomnia is defined as the inability to obtain sufficient sleep, or difficulty in falling or staying asleep. It is a risk factor for the onset of depression, and can negatively affect an individual's quality of life. A healthy lifestyle can often help to manage insomnia, but it does not eliminate the condition. Fortunately there are treatment options available for insomnia such as behavioral therapy, prescription medications, or a combination of the two. The most common practices of behavioral therapy are stimulus control, cognitive therapy, sleep restriction, and relaxation training. Behavioral therapy is conducted by a psychiatrist, psychologist, or counselor and focuses on ways to change behavior that may be contributing to poor sleep. Research has indicated that behavioral therapy is often more effective, and the positive outcomes last longer than those obtained through medication.

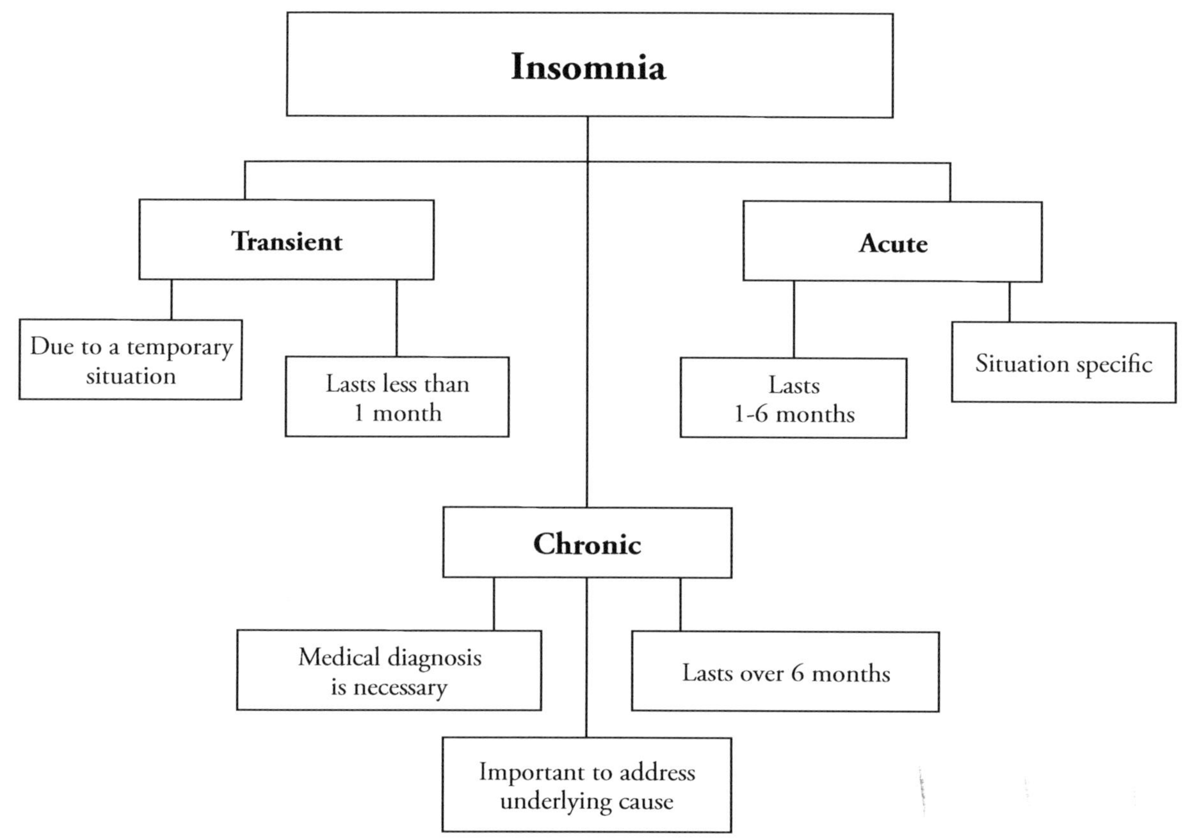

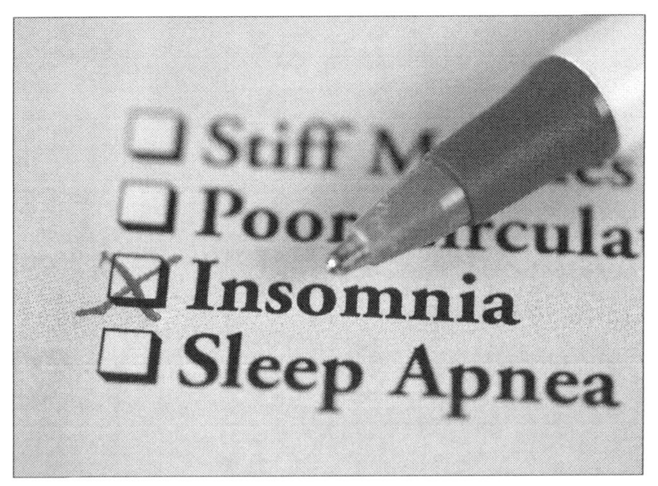

Insomnia can be classified as transient, acute, or chronic. Transient insomnia is the least severe case, lasting only one month or less, and is typically related to a specific situation such as stress at work or family problems.

Transient insomnia will diminish when the specific situation linked to the condition begins to improve or is no longer present. Acute insomnia is more severe than transient, lasting about 1-6 months, and is also related to a specific situation such as a stressful or emotional event. The difference between transient and acute insomnia is the length of time they last. Chronic insomnia is the most severe of the three conditions, lasting six months or longer. Generally, a medical diagnosis is necessary because there is usually a more serious health problem or other underlying cause.

Currently, there are approximately 100 different sleep disorders. The most prevalent disorders include sleep apnea, restless leg syndrome, and disruption of the circadian rhythm. Forty million Americans suffer from sleep disorders. Each year sleep disorders cost employers $60 billion in lost productivity, industrial accidents, and medical expenses. Sleep disorders affect the quality and quantity of a person's sleep. The discomfort and fatigue that results from sleep disorders is significant, and it varies with each person. Treatment for sleep disorders depends on the condition. In addition, good lifestyle habits, proper sleep hygiene practices, and the use of a sleep diary are helpful ways to alleviate some of the discomforts associated with sleep disorders.

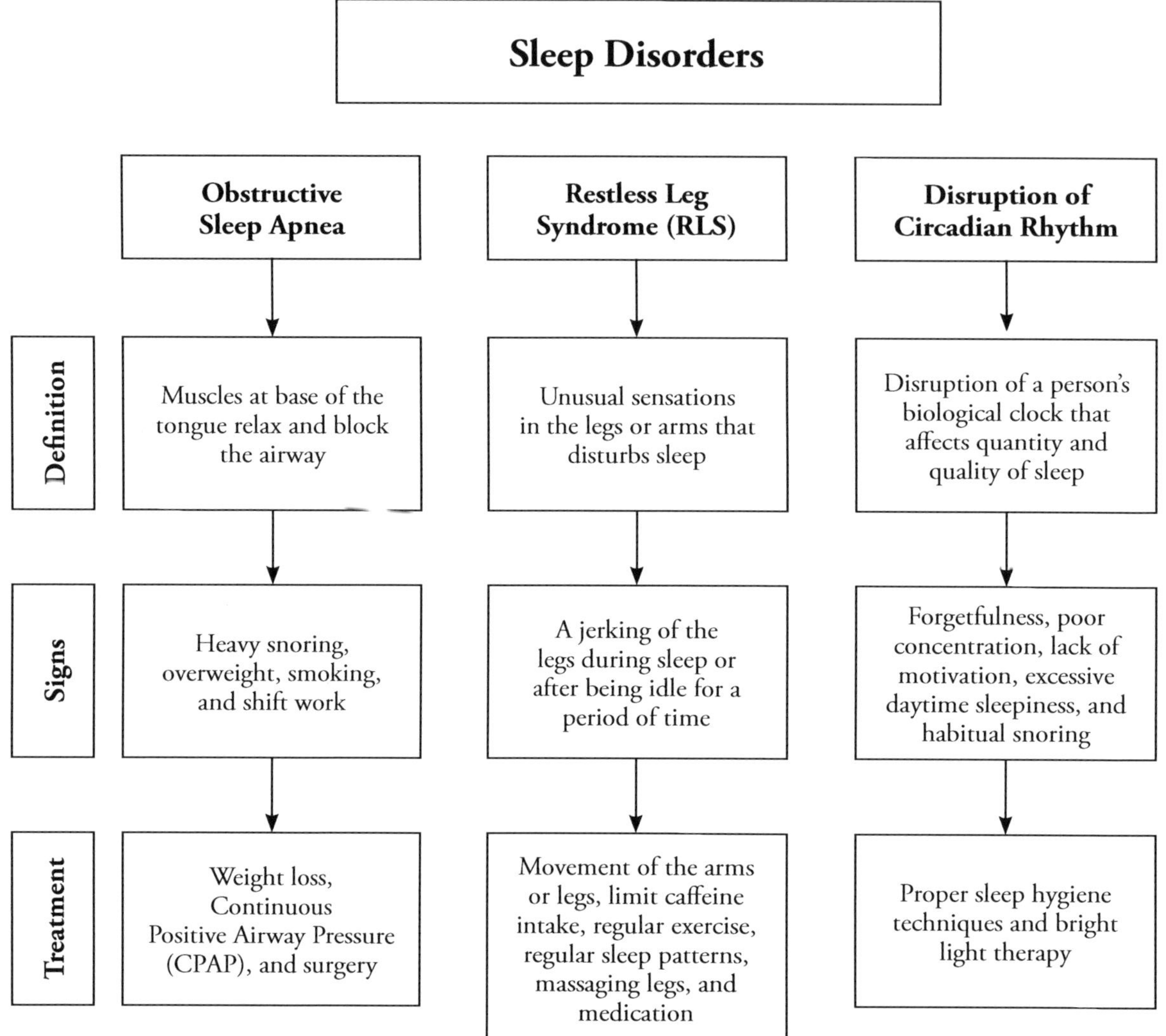

Sleep Apnea

There are various sleep disorders. However, sleep apnea, Restless Leg Syndrome (RLS), and disruption of the circadian rhythm are among the most common. Central apnea is a form of sleep apnea caused by problems with how the brain controls breathing, rather than a blockage of the throat as in obstructive sleep apnea. Central apnea is not the most common form of sleep apnea. Research has indicated there may be an association between Sudden Infant Death Syndrome (SIDS) and central apnea. The most severe of the sleep disorders is obstructive sleep apnea.

Obstructive sleep apnea affects 18 million Americans. One example occurs when the individual is sleeping and the muscles at the base of the tongue and the uvula (the small piece of tissue that hangs down at the back of your throat) relax and sag. This blocks the airway for a short time, causing the sleeper to begin to thrash around as they struggle to get back to regular breathing. While the sleeper is unaware of what is happening during sleep, they will begin to feel the effects of their impaired rest, which can impact work performance. Obstructive sleep apnea can also occur due to improper jaw alignment or tonsils/adenoids obstructing the airway.

Sleep apnea typically occurs in people who are overweight. The excess neck tissue narrows the airway. Even though individuals may not be aware of their condition, there are specific signs and risks to indicate a person may have or be at risk for obstructive sleep apnea. These signs include breathing cessation, heavy snoring, excessive sleepiness during the day, or disturbance of bed partner. The risk factors associated include being a male between 40-60 or a female over 50 years of age, overweight/obesity, cigarette smoking, and alcohol use.

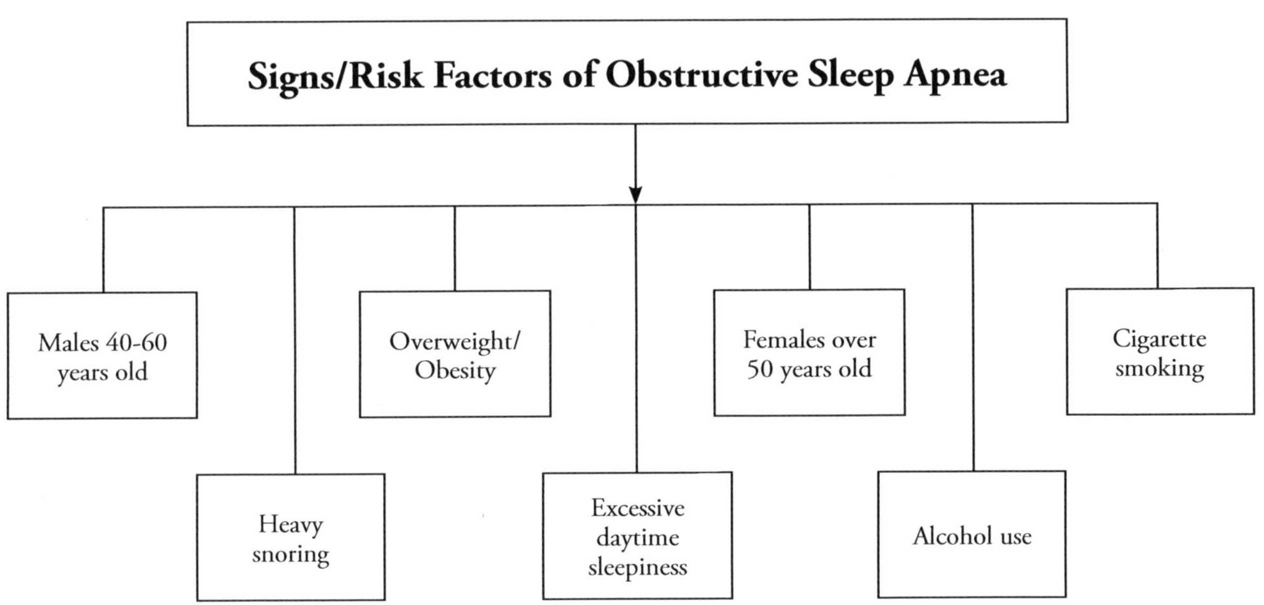

The good news about this disorder is that it can be treated with weight loss, Continuous Positive Airway Pressure (CPAP), surgery, or jaw alignment. Weight loss can help reduce the number of waking episodes when a person reduces their weight by only 10%. Continuous Positive Airway Pressure is delivered by a mask worn at night, and is attached to a device that forces air through the nose to keep the tissue in the throat from collapsing. Surgery involves the removal of the excess tissue from the uvula and other areas to prevent collapsing of the airways. Lastly, jaw alignment, which involves tongue-retaining devices or bite guards, can be used to bring the lower jaw forward and thereby alleviate airway obstruction during sleep. If you think you have symptoms of obstructive sleep apnea it is important to consult your doctor or a certified sleep specialist as soon as possible.

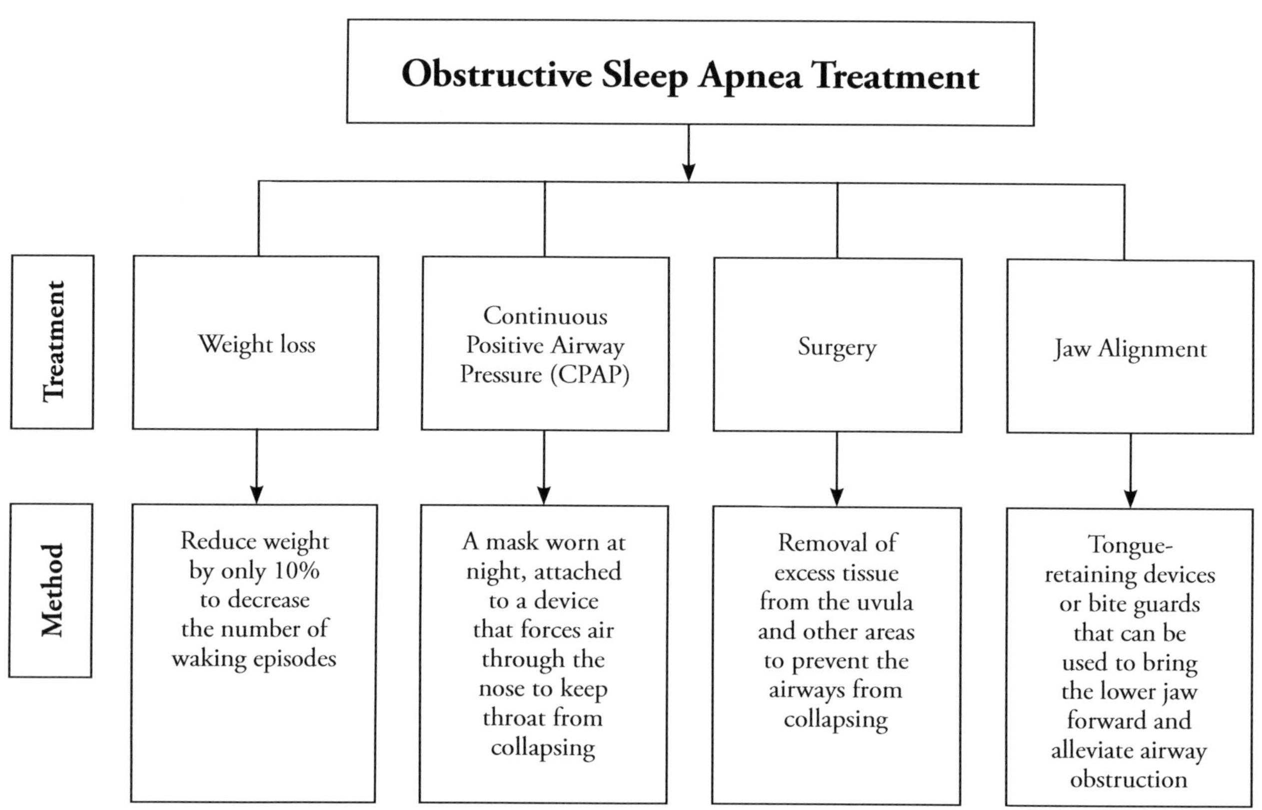

Restless Leg Syndrome (RLS)

Restless Leg Syndrome (RLS) is a neurological condition caused by a tingling sensation in the extremities, usually the legs. This disorder causes an individual to have an uncontrollable urge to move their legs, often resulting in sleep disturbance or trouble falling asleep. Symptoms of RLS tend to become worse the longer a person is idle, or when resting. The symptoms of RLS also worsen in the evening. The only way to relieve the sensations felt with this disorder is to move your legs or extremities. This condition often occurs during pregnancy, but it does affect both males and females. Many treatment options exist, but most involve preventive measures such as limiting caffeine intake, getting regular exercise, adhering to a regular sleep pattern, or massaging the legs. Medications are also available to treat symptoms of RLS.

Circadian Rhythm Disruption

There are two types of circadian rhythm disruption, advanced and delayed (happens in younger individuals). Disruption of the circadian rhythm involves a person's biological clock. In this situation the clock runs later or earlier than the norm. This disruption affects the quality and quantity of sleep and often leads to insomnia or excessive sleepiness. This disorder can be secondary to other causes such as shift work, jet lag, daylight savings time, and varying work schedules. However, disruption of the circadian rhythm can also be a primary disorder not associated with other causes. Often, individuals will experience forgetfulness, poor concentration, lack of motivation, excessive daytime sleepiness, and habitual snoring as a result of this disruption. Common treatment options for this disorder include proper sleep hygiene techniques, bright light therapy designed to reset the person's circadian rhythm, and chronobiology - where sleep times and durations are varied using forward rotation.

While there are treatment options available for fatigue and insomnia, such as medication and behavioral therapy, there is also an array of prevention strategies available. Before expensive medications and visits to a therapist, psychiatrist, or psychologist, these prevention strategies are lifestyle changes you can make on your own or with the help of a health coach. Some tips to help overcome insomnia and fatigue include waking up at the same time every day if possible; avoiding alcohol, caffeine, and nicotine before bed; exercising (but not within three hours of going to bed); sleeping in a dark, quiet, and cool room; and using a sleep diary to record sleep patterns and problems. Napping is also helpful, especially for shift workers, to help supplement sleep. However, napping may be contraindicative for those who suffer from insomnia or other sleep disorders because it may reinforce erratic sleeping patterns that already exist, so it is important to consult with your doctor.

Tips to Overcome Insomnia and Fatigue

Environment Concerns
- » Stick to a routine when traveling
- » Use bed for sleep only
- » Wake up at the same time daily

Bedtime Rituals
- » Take a warm bath
- » Use relaxation techniques
- » Set the room temperature to be comfortable

Light
- » Use the curtains or blinds to keep the room dark
- » Wear eyeshades
- » Avoid light when possible

Food
- » No caffeine four to five hours before bed
- » Avoid alcohol
- » Eat a light snack before bed if hungry

Exercise
- » Reduce stress by regular exercise
- » Do not exercise less than 3 hours before bed

Sleep Diary
- » Useful to describe sleep patterns and symptoms
- » Be aware of what works for you

Life and Work Balance
- » Talk to friends and family about your concerns
- » Do not take out irritability from sleep loss on friends, family, or co-workers

Napping
- » Take 20-minute naps
- » A 1-5 minute nap may result in feeling refreshed
- » Important for those who work double shifts or 24-hour shifts
- » Careful consideration if sleep disorders are present

Alertness at work (shift workers)
- » Take adequate breaks if possible
- » Be physically active during breaks
- » Talk with co-workers to help you stay alert
- » Do not drink caffeine prior to bedtime

The "Tips to overcome Insomnia and Fatigue" schematic offers alternatives to typical treatment options. Through simple lifestyle changes an individual may be able to alleviate the severity of their fatigue and/or insomnia. It is not necessary to adapt all of the practices, instead implement the strategies that work best for you and stick with them. Repetition is important because it allows your body to become accustomed to your new lifestyle changes and gradually helps to lessen your symptoms.

Sleep Myths

There have always been common myths associated with sleep. Many people believe that turning on the radio or the air conditioner in the car will help them to stay awake. Others believe that lying in bed, tossing and turning, will eventually lead to them falling sleep. These common misconceptions are not only wrong, but they can be harmful to your sleep patterns and dangerous to your health.

The "Common Sleep Myths" schematic illustrates common sleep myths and identifies the facts surrounding each. For example, believing that turning on the air conditioner, turning up the radio, or opening a window will help prevent a tired driver from falling asleep is a dangerous myth. The only thing that will safely and effectively prevent a tired driver from falling asleep is 15-45 minute nap in a safe rest area. Research has indicated that a combination of napping and strategically used caffeine consumption will help a sleepy individual become more alert. However, it is important to note that naps may further contribute to erratic sleep patterns in those who suffer from insomnia and other sleep disorders. Another myth is related to the amount of sleep older adults think they require; you often hear claims that adults need less sleep as they age. However, it is the sleep pattern that changes, and not the amount of sleep needed. In fact, older adults tend to get less sleep at night, but take more naps throughout the day due to less deep and more fragmented sleep.

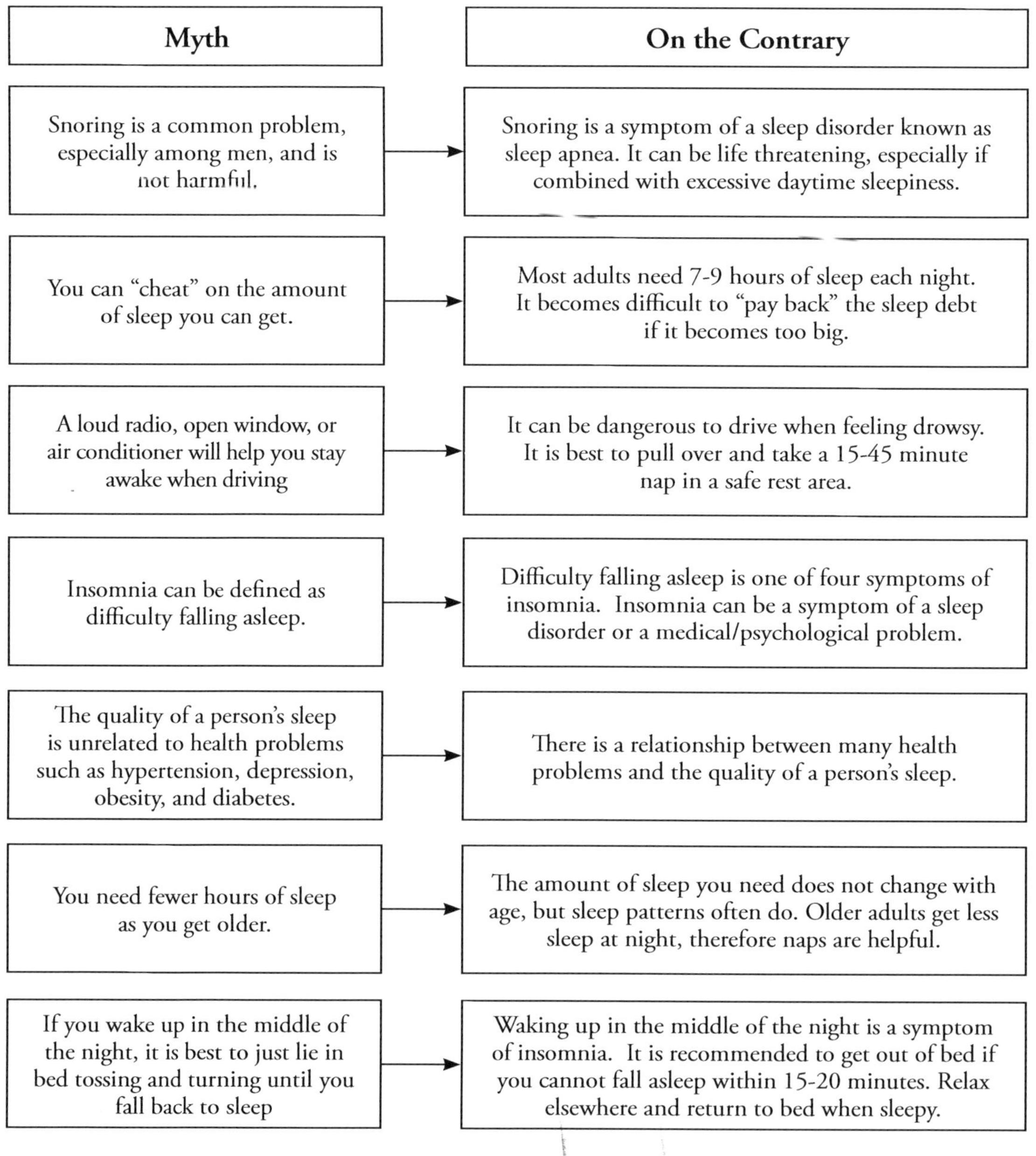

Sleep needs change with age. A newborn and an adolescent vary greatly on the amount of sleep they need. Even the amount of sleep needed for a 25 year old will be quite different from the sleep needs of an elderly adult. It is crucial to realize your sleep needs because your quality of sleep greatly affects how you feel and perform. However, there is no "magic number" for the amount of sleep needed by each individual. Due to the highly individualized nature of sleep, everyone is different regarding how much sleep they need to perform each day.

Sleep Needs Throughout The Life Cycle	
Infants and Babies	
0 – 2 months	10.5 – 18.5 hours
2 – 12 months	14 – 15 hours
Toddlers and Children	
12 – 18 months	13 – 15 hours
18 months – 3 years	12 – 14 hours
3 – 5 years	11 – 13 hours
5 – 12 years	9 – 11 hours
Adolescents	
13 – 18 years	8.5 – 9.5 hours
Adults	
Over 18 years	7 – 9 hours (on average)

There are many factors that may affect the quality and quantity of your sleep. Often lifestyle and overall health affect sleep patterns, leading to fatigue or sleep disorders. It is important for each person to assess what lifestyle factors may be affecting them so they can get the sleep they need to perform daily tasks at work and home. Fortunately, when life becomes too stressful and the right amount of sleep is not an option, there are simple lifestyle changes you can make to help prevent fatigue, such as the strategies previously discussed.

Chapter 2 – Sleep Hygiene – Why is it important?

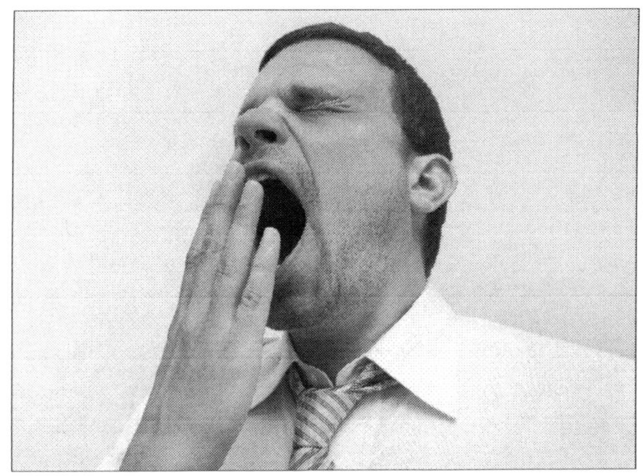

In today's fast-paced society where email, cell phones, Internet, and television continue to evolve and present new ways to stimulate, there has emerged a growing problem of voluntary sleep reduction. As the prevalence of sleep disorders, insomnia, and societal/cultural pressures continue to increase sleep reduction, the need for good sleep hygiene practices is greater than ever before as a preventive measure for fatigue. The rationale behind sleep hygiene is to improve sleep quality.

Sleep hygiene involves practices or strategies that are essential for normal, quality sleep during your down time and alertness during work or wake hours. Sleep hygiene also consists of behavioral practices that have been recognized to promote good rest. Good sleep hygiene is important because it helps prevent the development of sleep disorders, and improves sleep quality. Practicing good sleep hygiene habits is the core strategy for several multi-component treatments of insomnia. Proper sleep hygiene practices leave an individual feeling more awake and alert throughout their waking hours.

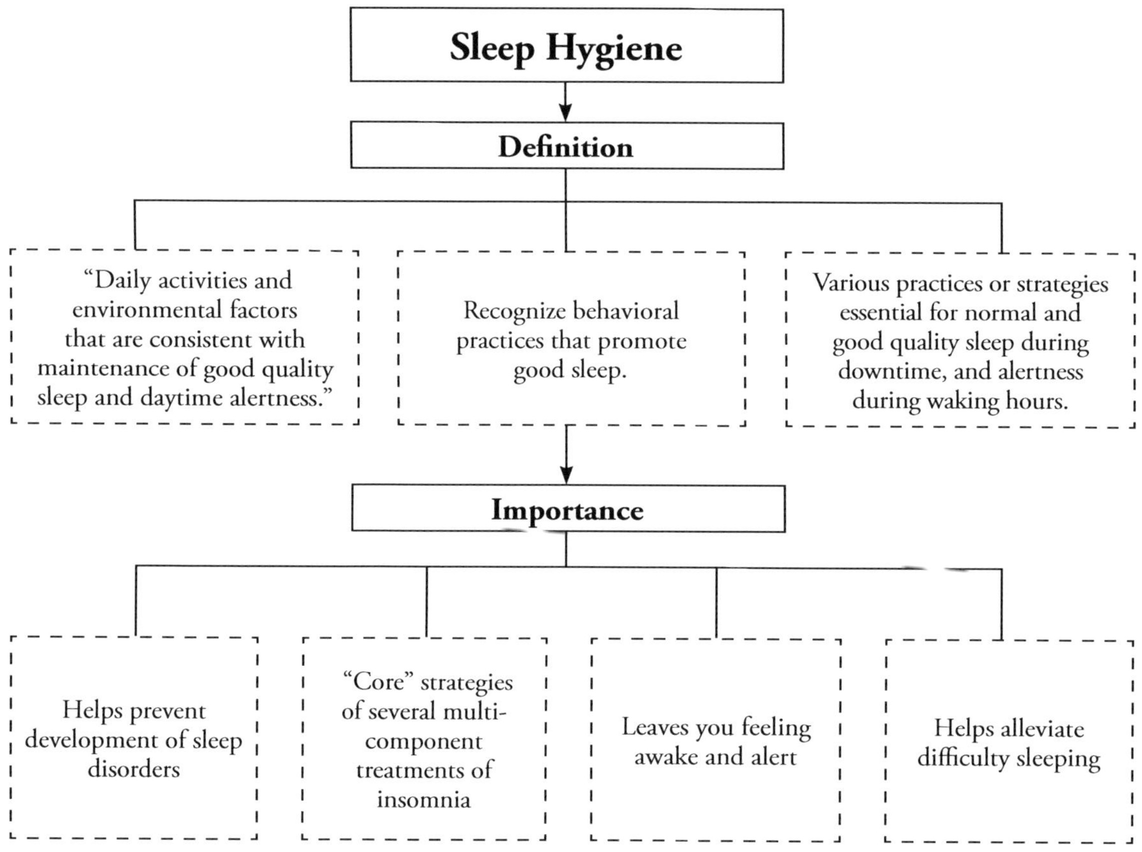

Even though good sleep hygiene is a crucial aspect to feeling rested and alert throughout waking hours, individuals still do not regularly practice it. Research has demonstrated a weak relationship between sleep practices and sleep hygiene knowledge. In other words, people do not take necessary action even though they 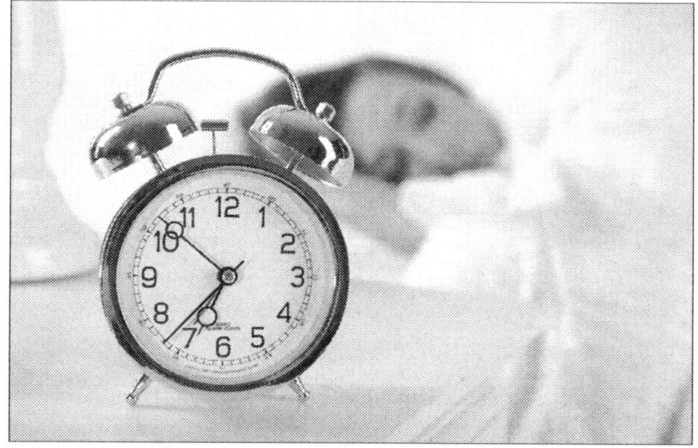 know what proper sleep hygiene practices are. This may be due to greater variation in sleep schedules from our fast-paced society. Unfortunately, there are several reasons why sleep hygiene or proper sleep habits are not practiced, which contribute to a greater incidence of insomnia.

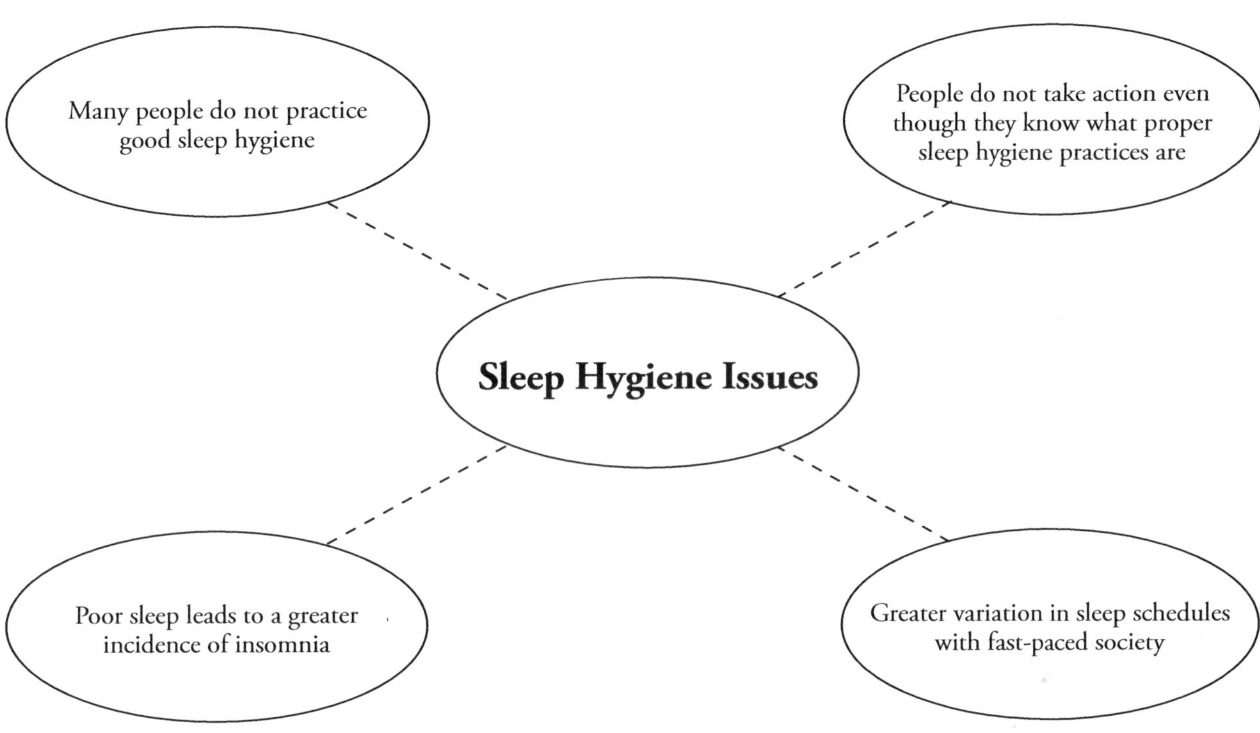

While there are many factors that affect proper sleep hygiene practices, there are various strategies that can be helpful. Often individuals perform bedtime rituals that may prevent them from sleeping, or cause them to have trouble falling asleep. Some examples include watching television in bed, or taking long naps throughout the day (unless you are a shift worker and you are napping to supplement sleep). Fortunately, there are strategies individuals can include in their lifestyle to assist with problems related to insomnia and other sleep disorders.

Strategies for better sleep hygiene include maintaining a regular sleep pattern seven days a week, if possible, depending on your work schedule, using your bed for sleeping only, avoiding heavy snacks and overeating before bedtime, limiting liquids and avoiding caffeine late before going to sleep, not exercising for at least three hours before going to sleep, taking naps for no longer than 20 minutes throughout the day (unless napping to supplement sleep), and avoiding alcohol and nicotine. Each of these strategies for sleep hygiene will be briefly discussed.

One of the primary strategies not commonly practiced is maintaining a regular sleep and wake pattern throughout the week. A person should go to bed and wake up at the same time every day, if possible, depending on your work schedule. This may help avoid sleep difficulties by regulating the circadian rhythm; getting mind and body used to sleeping at a specific time. Using your bed for sleep only; and avoiding television, eating, or doing work in your bed is another helpful tip. This helps associate the bed with sleep. When you watch television or do work in bed you begin to associate your bed with being awake, or perhaps with a stressful situation that may affect your sleep.

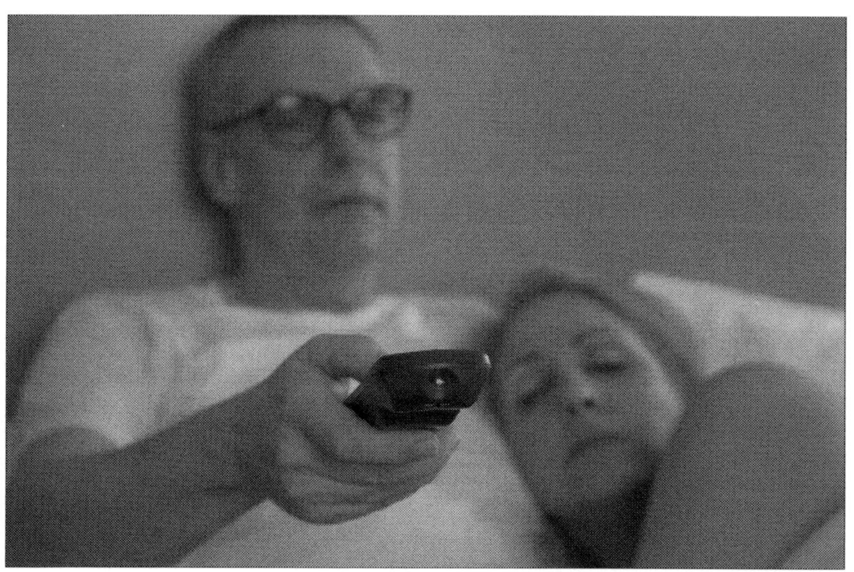

Exercising less than three hours before bedtime can also prevent good sleep. Some people believe that exercise will make them feel tired and help them sleep better, but if done too close to bedtime exercise can leave you feeling more alert and awake. While exercise does help you to sleep better, doing it too close to the time you plan to sleep may be counterproductive. Exercise is not the only activity to avoid before bedtime. Ingesting caffeine, alcohol, and using products with nicotine should not be done near bedtime. Caffeine and nicotine are stimulants that can lead to feeling more awake. Alcohol, while it can make you feel sleepy, has adverse effects on sleep quality. Not smoking is a good idea for improved sleep, and for other health reasons as well. Napping throughout the day for longer than 20 minutes can affect a person's sleep as well. While naps do help to combat sleepiness, too long of a nap can leave you so well rested that you have trouble falling asleep at bedtime. This will begin to have an affect on your circadian rhythm, and lead to even more trouble sleeping. However, napping strategies should be used with erratic schedules or shift work. Lastly, overeating, eating heavy meals, or drinking too many liquids before bed will greatly affect a person's sleep. Bedtime or late night snacks do not have to be avoided, but should be limited to a light snack consisting of a carbohydrate or dairy product. Having a heavy meal right before bedtime may leave you feeling sick or uncomfortably full; this can adversely affect your sleep. Also, the amount of liquid a person drinks before going to sleep may interrupt sleep patterns. Drinking too much fluid may present the need to frequently urinate, disturbing sleep and making it hard to get back to sleep.

Each of the sleep hygiene strategies are depicted in the "Sleep Hygiene Strategies" schematic. While these strategies are designed to prevent sleep difficulties, all of the strategies may not be helpful. It may take time to identify which strategies are helpful for you, and which are not. By practicing good sleep hygiene strategies, and making them part of your lifestyle, you may be able to ensure good sleep patterns.

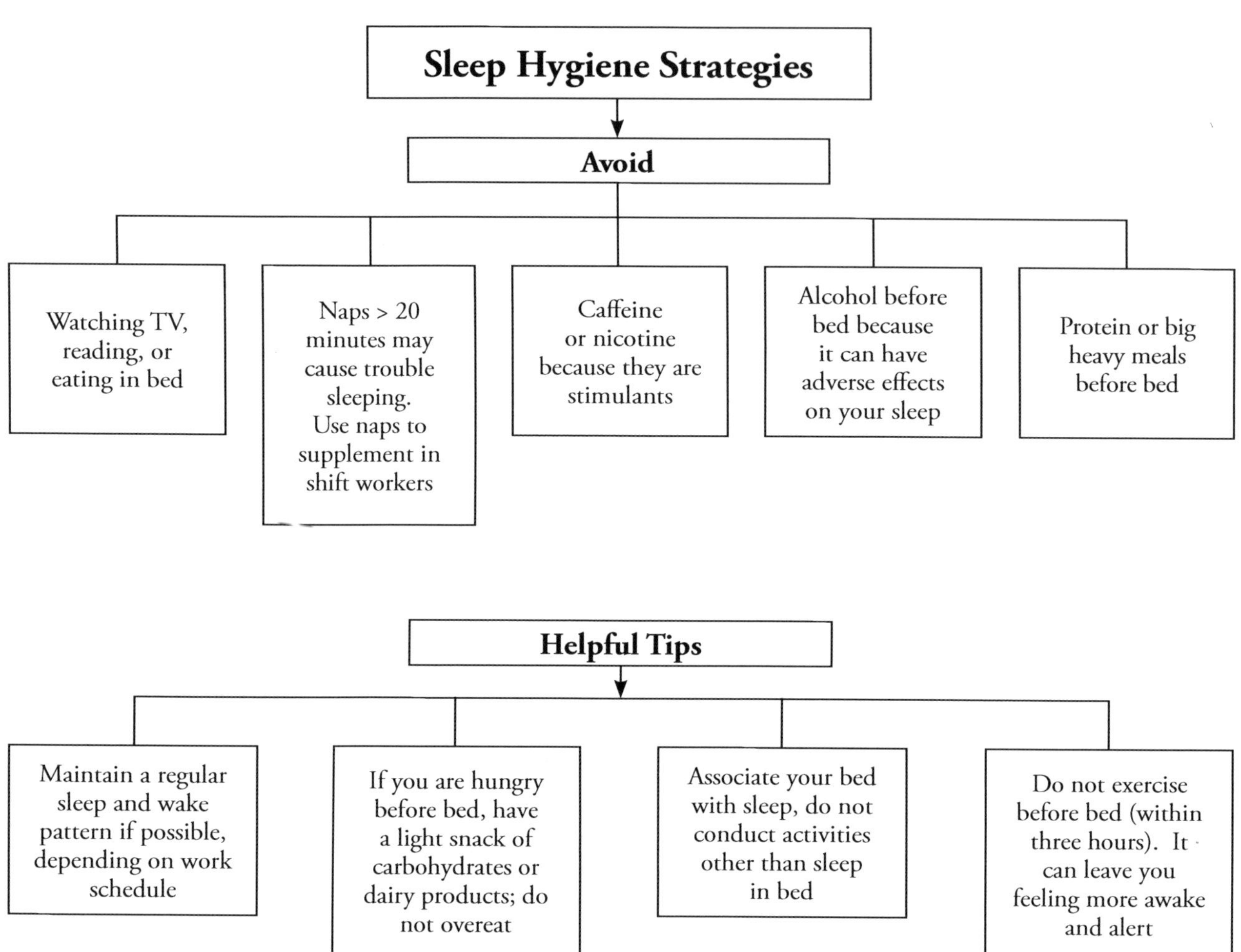
Sleep Hygiene Strategies
Avoid
Watching TV, reading, or eating in bed
Naps > 20 minutes may cause trouble sleeping. Use naps to supplement in shift workers
Caffeine or nicotine because they are stimulants
Alcohol before bed because it can have adverse effects on your sleep
Protein or big heavy meals before bed
Helpful Tips
Maintain a regular sleep and wake pattern if possible, depending on work schedule
If you are hungry before bed, have a light snack of carbohydrates or dairy products; do not overeat
Associate your bed with sleep, do not conduct activities other than sleep in bed
Do not exercise before bed (within three hours). It can leave you feeling more awake and alert

Often, the negative effects of improper sleep hygiene begin to influence the workplace. More employees are coming to work exhausted and at risk of falling asleep on the job. Fortunately for employers and employees there are actions that can be taken to make the workplace safe.

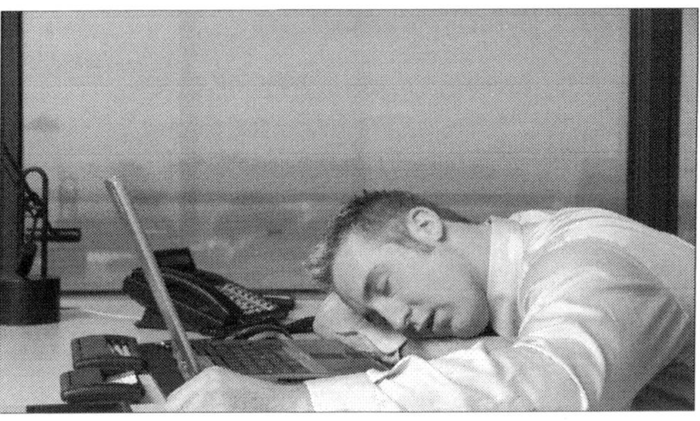

Good sleep hygiene is crucial to maintaining a sleep and wake schedule that leaves the person feeling alert and awake throughout the day. Without the use of positive sleep hygiene practices, the occurrence of insomnia and other sleep disorders may rise. In a fast-paced society, sleep hygiene has become imperative for a good rest. As you know, there are various strategies within the workplace and at home to help combat excessive sleepiness. With the help of these strategies, and a few lifestyle changes, most individuals will be able to increase their quality of life and be alert throughout the day.

Chapter 3 – Stress

For many people, stress is a part of their everyday lives. It may be caused by an illness, a personal problem, or running late for work. However, what is perceived as a stressful situation by one individual may not be for someone else. Stress is defined as "the inability to cope with a threat (real or imagined) to your well-being, which results in a series of responses and adaptations by your body." Stress can affect you in many ways: physically, cognitively, emotionally, and/or behaviorally. There are many different stressors: internal, external, distress (bad), eustress (good), and occupational. These stressors and symptoms will be discussed in greater detail later in this chapter. The schematic below provides an overview of stress.

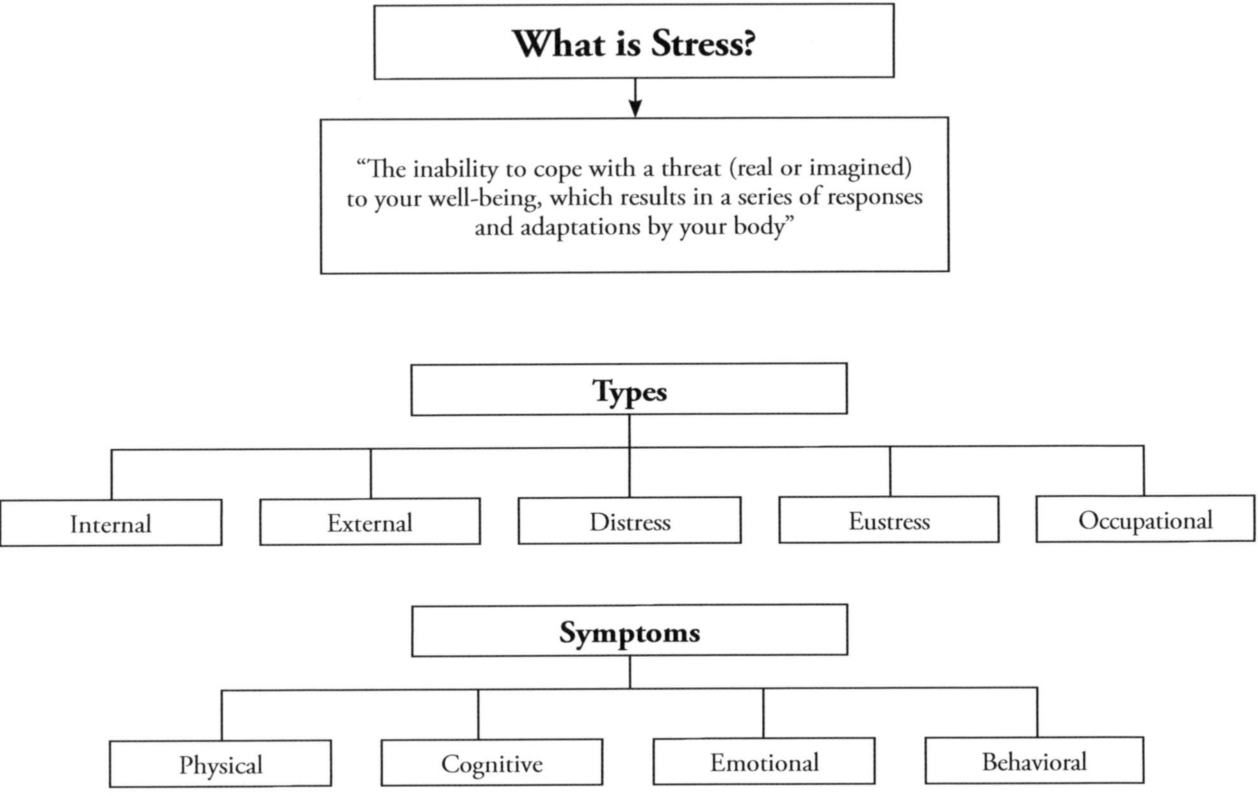

Stress has a vast affect on the workplace. One million employees miss work everyday due to stress, which results in $300 billion lost annually. Approximately 25% of employees listed their job as their number one stressor, while 40% said their job is extremely stressful. Stress contributes to physical ailments and sickness for 36% of workers, while 44% of women and 36% of men want to quit their jobs because of workplace stress. Even though stressors are everywhere, it should be no surprise that employees report stress at work.

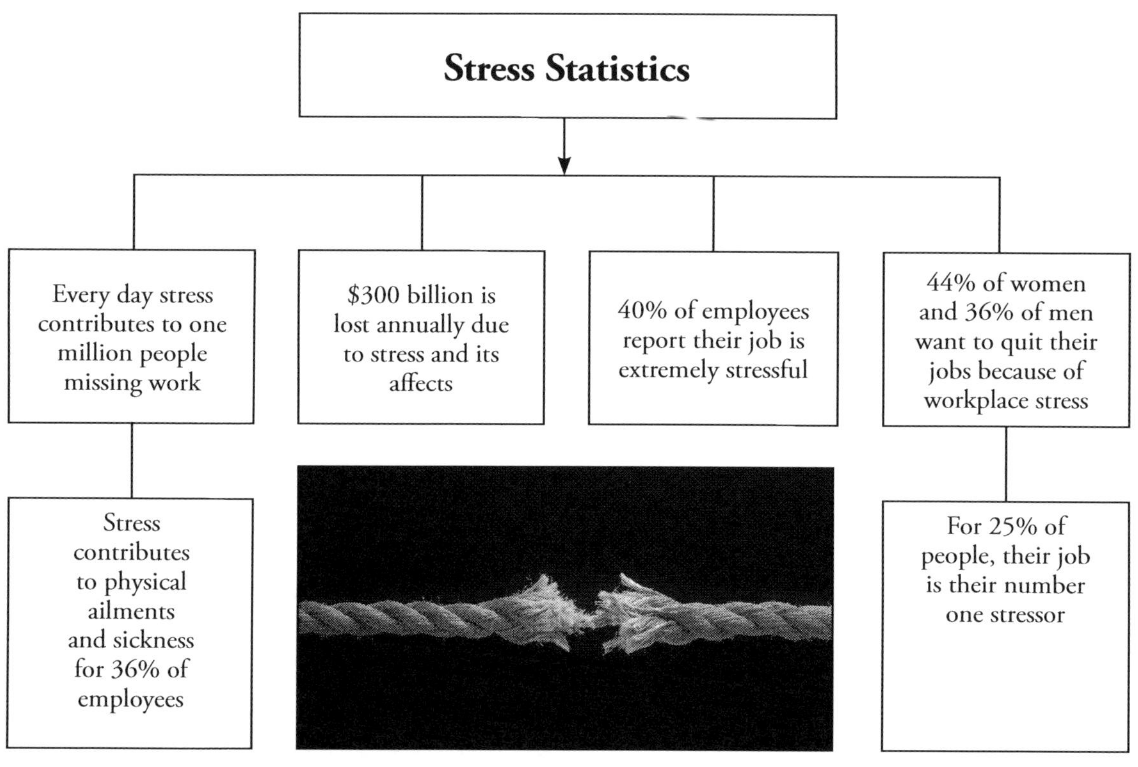

While workplace or occupational stress can have an effect on an individual's performance, there are other stressors that also affect a person's perception of their stress level. Stressors include: internal, external, distress, eustress, and occupational. Internal stress involves personal emotion or activities. This stress can result from poor nutrition, too much or no physical activity, lack of spiritual fulfillment, or personal interests. External stress comes from the outside environment including noise, air pollution, overcrowding, negative personal interactions, heavy traffic, or major life changes. Internal and external stressors are considered either good stress (eustress) or bad stress (distress). It is important to remember not all stress will negatively affect a person. For example, eustress creates excitement and happiness. Depending on an individual's outlook or perception, the following may cause eustress: getting a job promotion, having a child, holidays, a child going to college, or graduations. These stressors are seen as positive events in a person's life. However, there are also things that lead to distress - the type of stress most people think of when they think of stress. Distress typically has a negative affect on a person, and can either be acute or chronic depending on the situation. Distress arises from many events such as divorce, death of a family member or loved one, unemployment, financial difficulties, pressure to perform at work, or drug/alcohol abuse.

Another stressor is occupational stress. It can be a combination of any of the stressors previously discussed (internal, external, eustress, or distress) depending on the situation. Typically, occupational stress can be defined as, "harmful physical and emotional responses that can happen when there is a conflict between job demands on the employee and the amount of control an employee has over meeting those demands." This stress may occur when events take place such as, job promotions or demotions, strained co-worker relationships, financial instability, increased responsibility, shift work or long hours, and conflicting management styles.

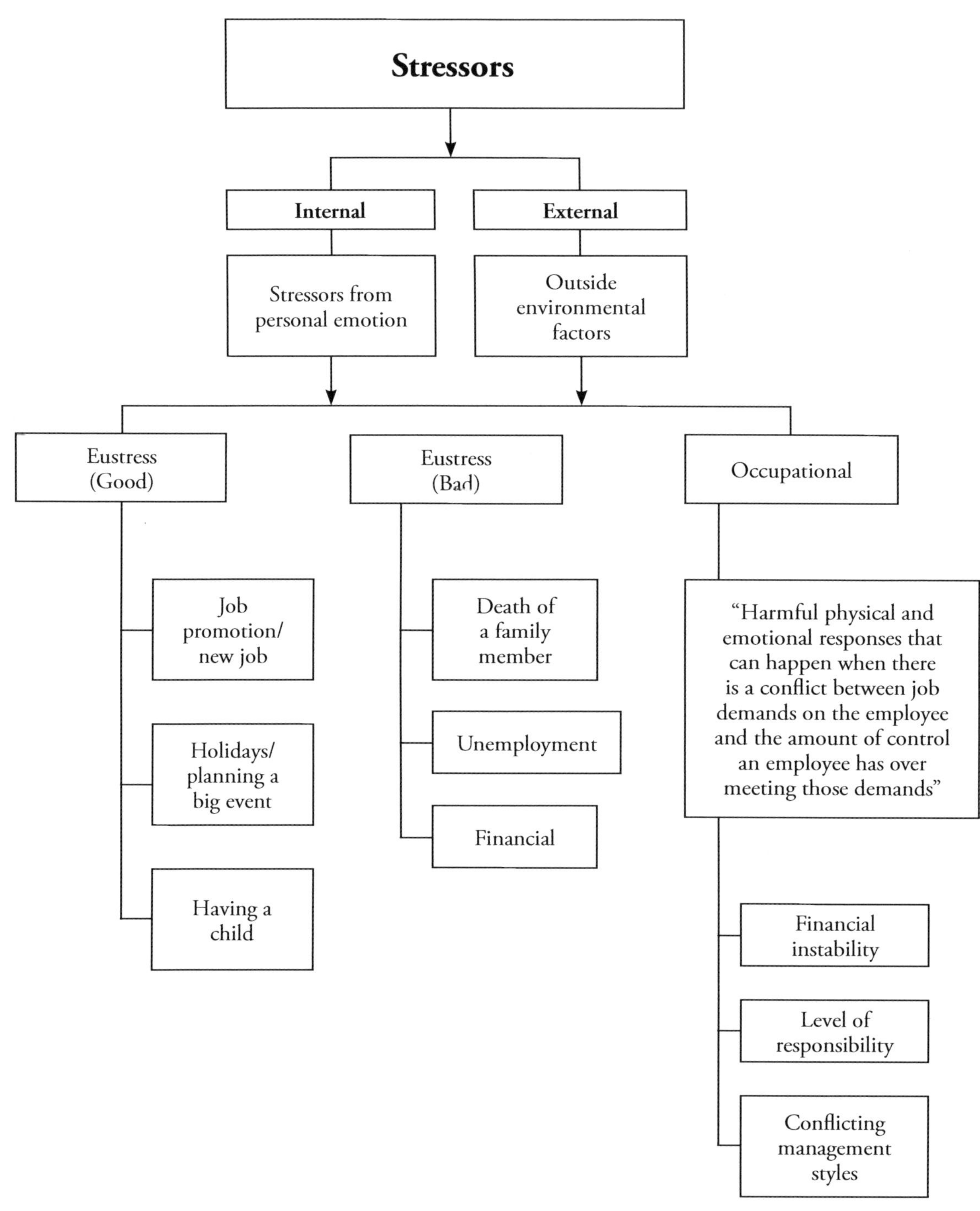

Stressors
Internal
External
Stressors from personal emotion
Outside environmental factors
Eustress (Good)
Eustress (Bad)
Occupational
Job promotion/ new job
Holidays/ planning a big event
Having a child
Death of a family member
Unemployment
Financial
"Harmful physical and emotional responses that can happen when there is a conflict between job demands on the employee and the amount of control an employee has over meeting those demands"
Financial instability
Level of responsibility
Conflicting management styles

Occupational stress is the primary source of stress for millions of Americans. Everyday you are faced with deadlines, projects, or meetings. It is your perception of those stressors and your ability to cope with them that contribute to your stress at work. Fortunately, there are various coping strategies for occupational stress: look back and recall past experiences, look into the future, realize you cannot control everything, talk freely with co-workers and management, and reduce personal conflicts. You should also take advantage of health improvement benefits, available personal leave or vacation time, and support options.

By looking back and recalling past experiences you are able to identify situations you have handled previously. This will allow you to remember your thoughts and feelings at the time which lead to the action taken. Recall the problem and how you handled it; be specific. Identify the results that occurred and if the outcome was positive or negative. This will help you handle your current or future situations so you receive the desired outcomes.

Realizing you cannot control all aspects of your life will help to reduce stress. So often, people focus on what they cannot change rather than what they can. It is important to identify what you do and do not have control over, and focus on the things you can control. By continuing to focus on things beyond your control, you may end up causing yourself more stress.

The coping techniques of speaking freely with co-workers and management and reducing personal conflicts are strategies that can be interrelated at times. Each technique is designed to open the lines of communication so you know what is expected of you. Allowing everyone to speak freely in a respectful manner, and offering suggestions and ideas can help to create a healthy and productive work environment.

Taking your scheduled vacations/personal time to recharge and relax can greatly help to reduce stress in the workplace. If possible, walking during lunch time or scheduled breaks can also help you feel more energized and calm your perception of stress.

Using available support such as your company's employee assistance program, local mental health providers, or various support groups can help you cope with stressful events. These options can provide you with therapeutic and positive outlets to express your concerns.

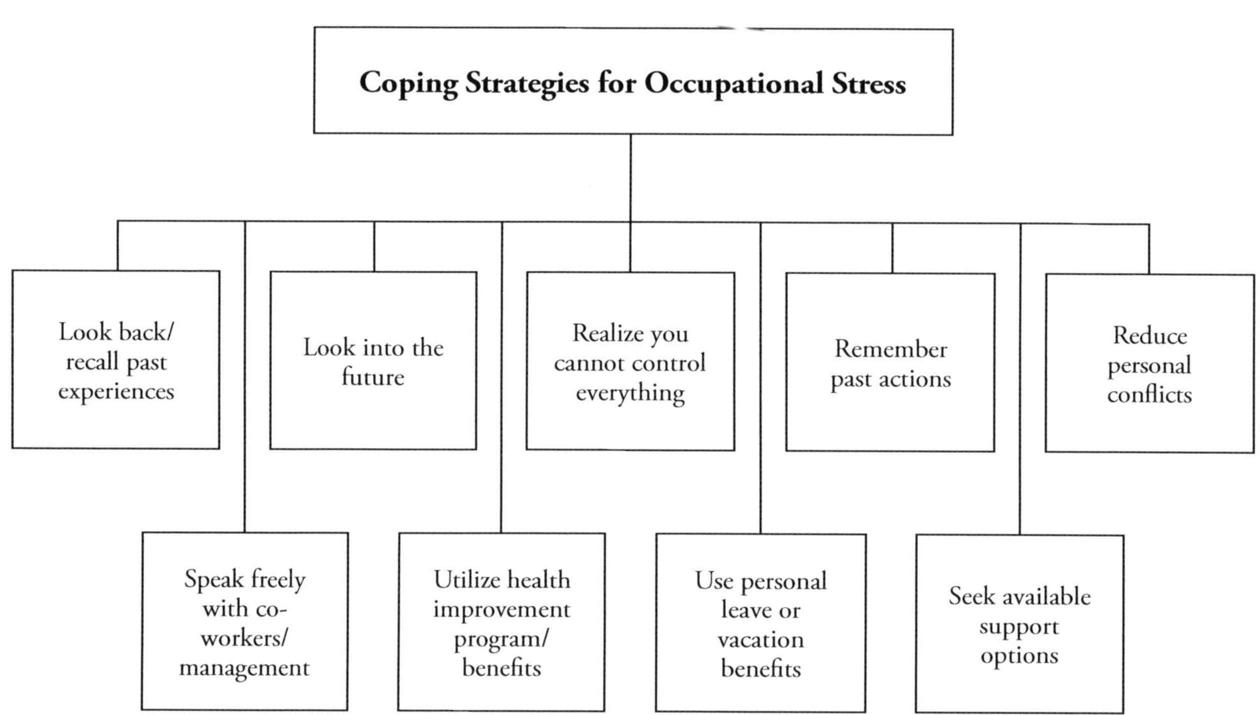

Stress affects each person differently. Some people may not experience any symptoms while others may experience headaches/migraines, depression, mood changes, or loss of appetite. Symptoms depend on the stressors and how long they last. As mentioned earlier in this chapter, stress symptoms fall into one of four categories: physical, cognitive, emotional, or behavioral. A person may experience symptoms from each category, or from just one or two. Symptoms associated with stress include headaches/migraines, depression, increase or decrease in appetite, high blood pressure, insomnia, nightmares or other trouble sleeping, poor concentration, and mood changes (such as irritation, anger, fear, panic, and anxiety). The Symptoms of Stress schematic identifies symptoms often associated with stress.

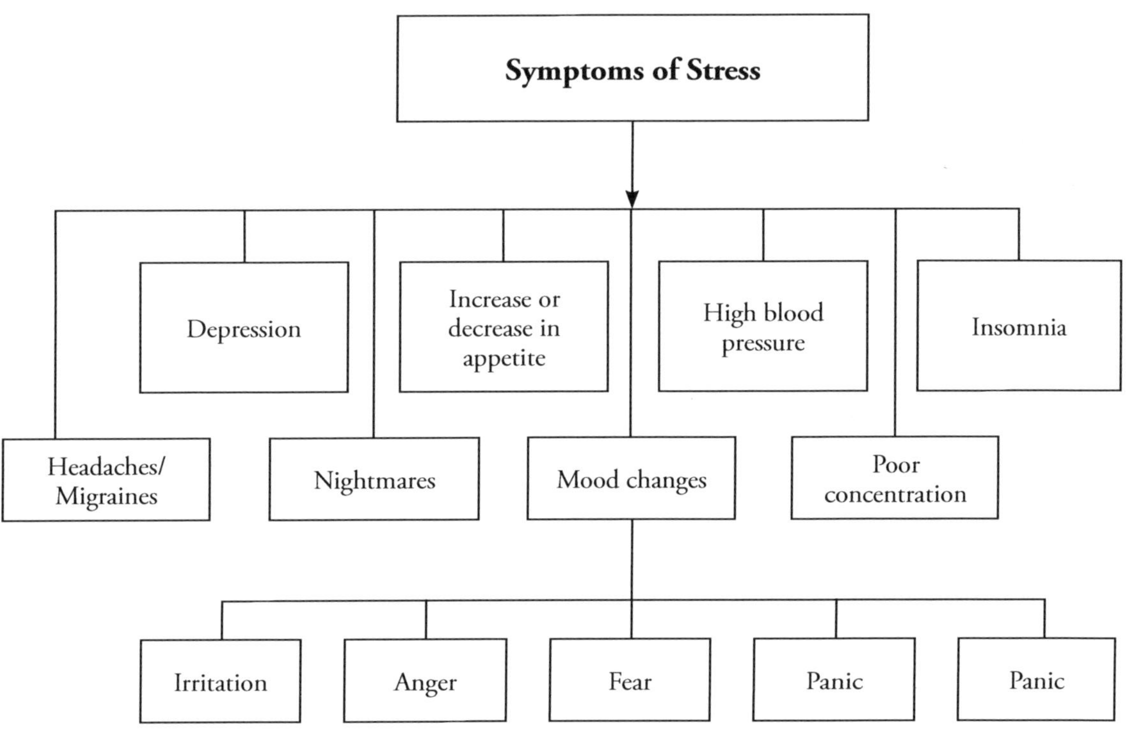

Stress is related to over 50% of all diseases, according to some experts. It is not the occasional stressful events, but chronic stress or continual stress that is linked to these diseases. Chronic stress can have a dramatic and harmful effect on your immune system, leading to poor health and even injury due to a lack of concentration. Chronic stress can lead to sleep disturbances, which negatively impact sleep patterns. There is also an increased vulnerability to insomnia caused by the perceived lack of control during stressful events. Stress is also linked to many other conditions: asthma, mental illness, suicide, ulcers, allergies, tooth decay, and high blood pressure. It is important to examine your stress levels, the underlying causes of your stress, and know what you can do to decrease your stress so you can avoid the negative affects.

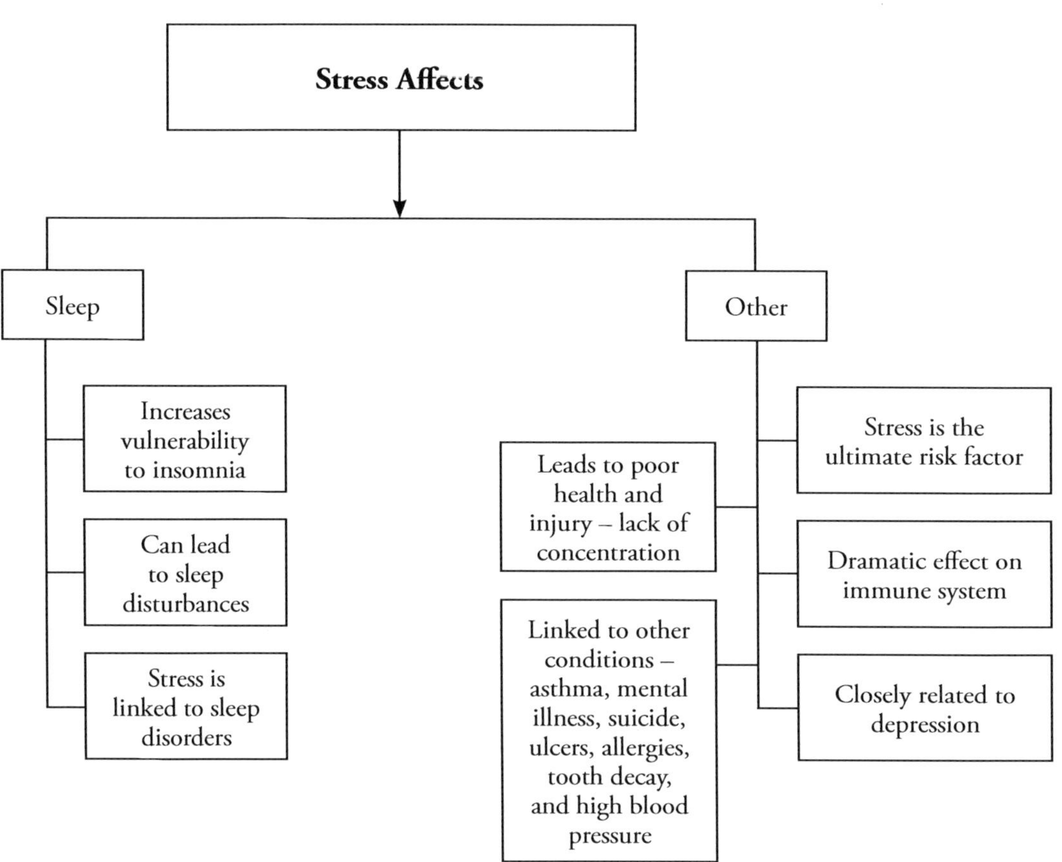

Stressors are everywhere. Stress cannot and should not be completely avoided. However, there are several strategies you can use to control stress and reduce its negative affects. These strategies include regular exercise, proper nutrition, stress relaxation techniques, adequate sleep, taking one thing at a time, managing your finances properly, enlisting social support, and practicing time management.

While each strategy helps reduce stress, they all provide relief in different ways. Exercising regularly can help reduce stress by providing an outlet, or time to decompress and relax. Exercise also serves as a way to reduce your risk for many diseases.

Proper nutrition, or increasing the intake of fruits and vegetables rather than eating unhealthy foods for comfort, is another stress-reducing strategy. Eating a healthy diet will give you energy needed to take on everyday stressors.

Practicing stress relaxation techniques such as meditation, deep breathing, yoga, and progressive muscle relaxation will help you channel stress in a positive manner. Stress relaxation techniques help you release distress and leave you feeling refreshed.

Because sleep disturbances are a negative result from stress, getting the appropriate amount of sleep is needed to combat possible sleep pattern disturbances. By maintaining a regular sleep pattern, when possible, you will be able to avoid daytime sleepiness and insomnia even during stressful times. If a regular sleep pattern is not always possible, using naps to supplement is also helpful.

Taking one thing at a time will allow you to feel less overwhelmed if tasks or projects start to pile up. This will allow you to look at the big picture so you can properly prioritize tasks.

Managing your finances will help reduce the burden of debt and monthly budget problems. Making payments on time and paying off debt can reduce stress.

Enlisting family, friends, and co-workers as a support system will provide you with an outlet to vent your stresses and daily concerns. Having social support will enable you to develop good relationships you can turn to in times of need or undue stress.

Practicing time management is related to schedule control and will help you identify the most important things in your life that need to get done. Time management will allow you to prioritize daily responsibilities and help you be more organized.

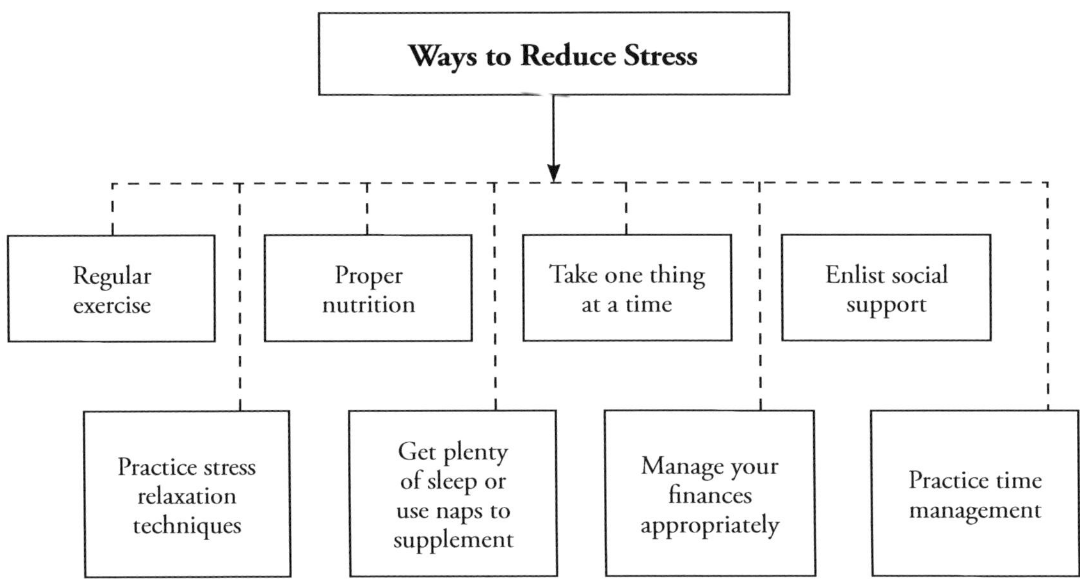

Stress does not have to be a negative influence in your life. It is essential to your well-being to realize your stressors, understand how your stressors affect you, and identify ways you can reduce or prevent personal distress. Remember that not all stress is bad, and your perception of things will determine how stress affects you, physically, mentally, emotionally, and behaviorally. By identifying your stressors and using appropriate coping strategies you will be better able to deal with stressful situations, allowing you to live a healthier and happier lifestyle.

Chapter 4 – Depression

For 18.8 million adults in the U.S., depression is an everyday obstacle. Depressive disorders are more than just a "blue mood" or a bad day. Depression affects all aspects of an individual's life: their body, mood, and thoughts. Depression affects the way a person eats, sleeps, feels about them self, thinks about things, and their overall view of the world around them. Often, there is a common misconception that people suffering from depression can simply 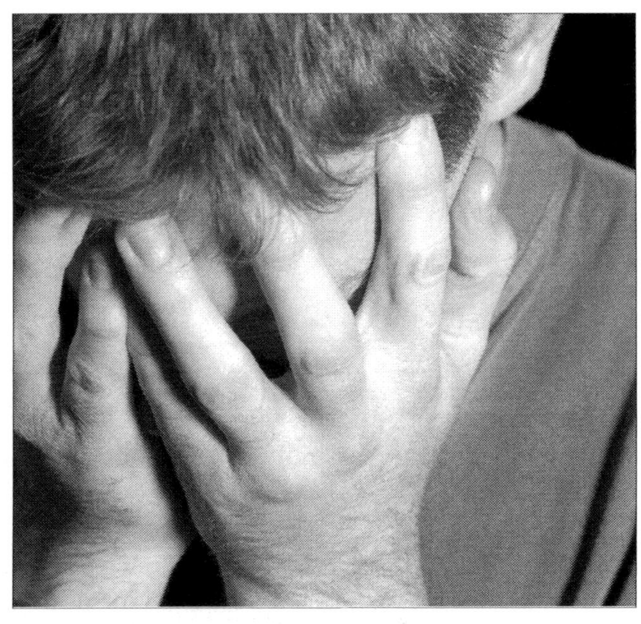 "pull themselves together" or "snap out of it." However, without proper treatment, the symptoms associated with depression can last for weeks, months, or even years.

Depression is defined as a medical illness that involves the body, mood, and thoughts. The major diagnoses of depression include major depression, dysthymia, and the bipolar disorders. Each depressive disorder varies by symptoms, severity, and persistence. Major depression is a combination of symptoms (i.e. feelings of hopelessness, guilt, and worthlessness, fatigue, and decreased appetite) that interfere with the ability to take part in daily activities. This depressive disorder often occurs several times throughout one's life.

Dysthymia is a less severe depressive disorder that involves the long-term chronic symptoms of depression, but does not disable a person. However, dysthymia does keep a person from feeling good and functioning well.

Bipolar disorders are a cycling between severe high (mania) and low (depression) moods, including gradual or dramatic and rapid mood shifts. Bipolar disorder is also called manic-depressive illness, and is not as prevalent as other depressive disorders. Bipolar I, Bipolar II, Cyclothymia, and Bipolar NOS are classifications of bipolar disorders.

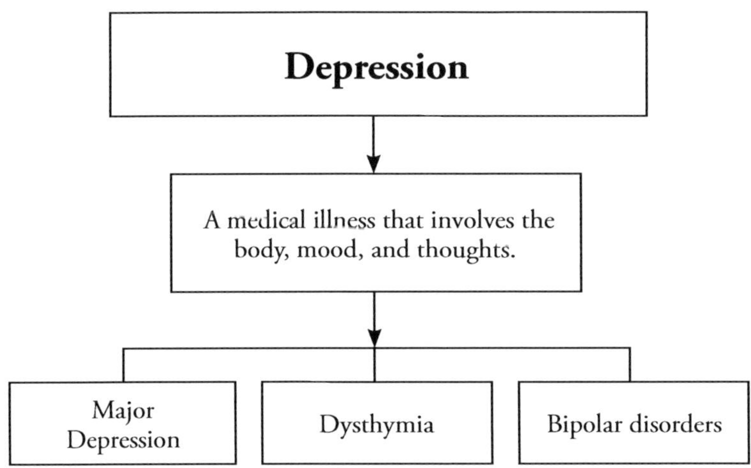

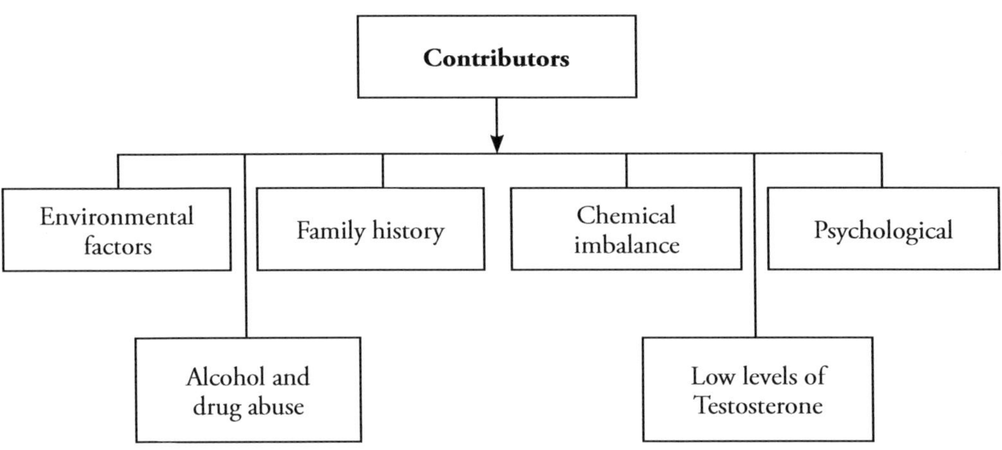

While depression rates are found to be similar between men and women, how it affects them is different. Men present symptoms differently than women. Men often hide their symptoms through drug and alcohol abuse, while women are more likely to report more "typical" depression symptoms and seek help. In addition, one out of ten men will be diagnosed with depression in their lifetime. The rate of suicide is four times higher in men, even though women attempt more suicides. This is because men choose more extreme measures than women, resulting in more successful suicide attempts. Sometimes in women, the cause of depression is hormonal such as menstrual cycle changes, pregnancy, miscarriage, pre-menopause, or menopause. Men suffer from a high death rate associated with the increased risk of coronary heart disease as a result of depression. The Depression Facts schematic provides statistics and facts related to depression.

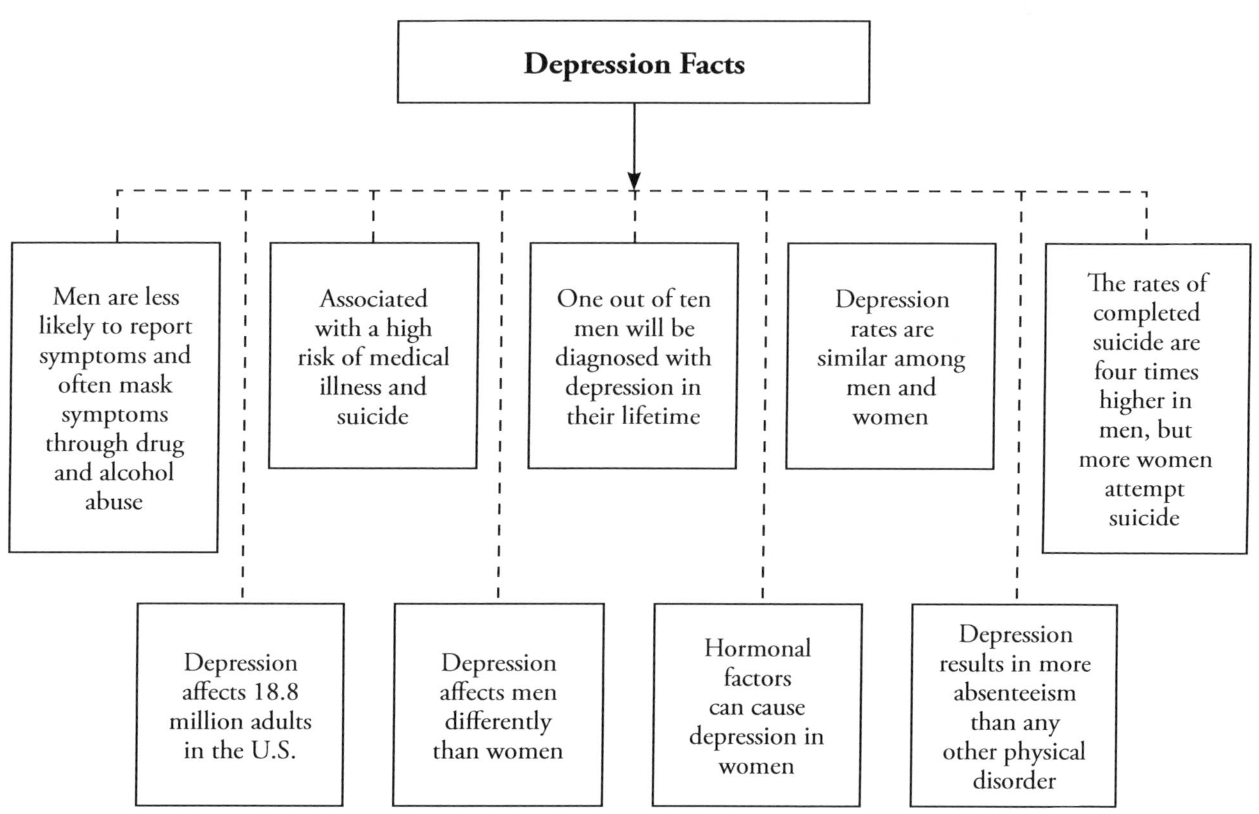

Not everyone who experiences depression will show symptoms. The specific symptoms a person experiences differs. Depending on the individual, the severity of the symptoms will vary. Time is also a factor since each individual will recover from depression at their own pace. Individuals suffering from depression may exhibit any one of the following symptoms: persistent sad, anxious, or "empty" mood; feelings of hopelessness, pessimism, guilt, worthlessness, or helplessness; loss of interest or pleasure in activities they once enjoyed; decreased energy or fatigue; difficulty concentrating, remembering, or making decisions; insomnia; decreased appetite and/or weight loss or overeating and/or weight gain; suicide attempts or thoughts of suicide; restlessness or irritability; or persistent physical symptoms that do not respond to treatment such as headaches.

Those suffering with depressive conditions that include manic features have some of the following symptoms, abnormal or excessive elation, unusual irritability, decreased need for sleep, grandiose notions, increased talking, racing thoughts, increased sexual desire, markedly increased energy, poor judgment, and inappropriate social behavior.

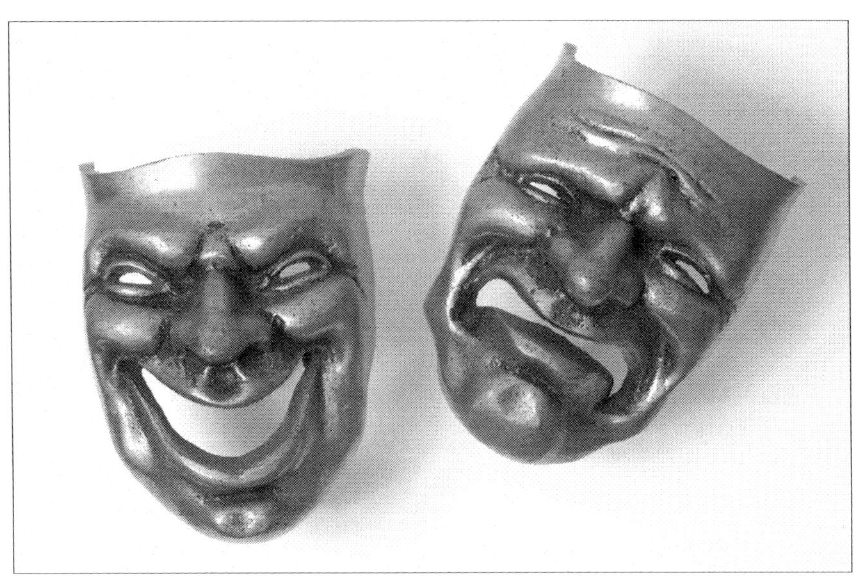

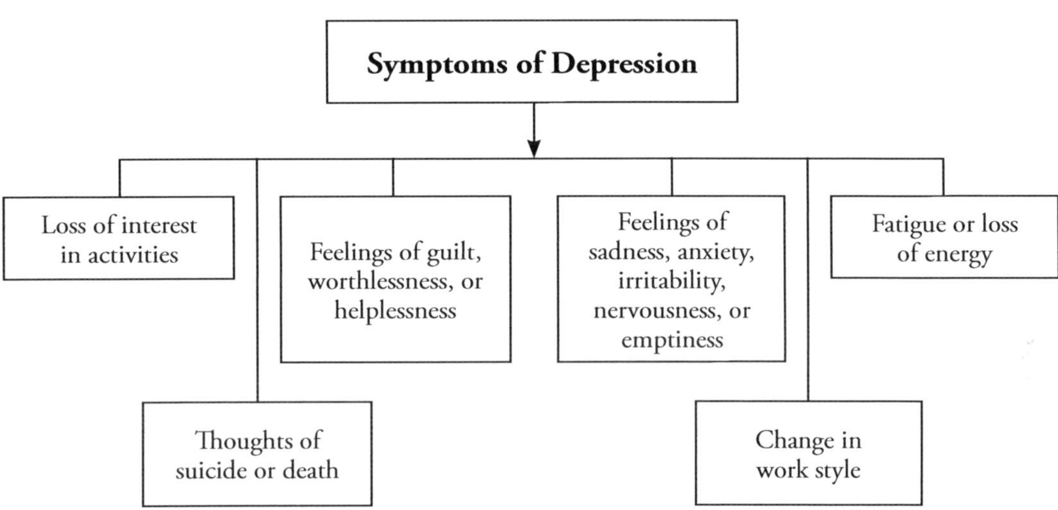

Typically everyone, at some time in their life, will be affected by depression. This could be depression of their own or that of someone close to them. Fortunately, there are many strategies or treatments that can help to address the symptoms of depression. The most common treatments are talk therapy, medication, and lifestyle changes.

Talk therapy is an effective treatment for depressive disorders. Talk therapy or psychotherapy can be provided by different health care professionals such as, psychologists, psychiatrist, social workers, and mental health counselors. Most often used methods include: behavioral, cognitive, Cognitive Behavioral Therapy (CBT), and interpersonal therapy. Behavioral therapy encourages changes in how the depressed person acts and responds. Cognitive therapy helps the individual to overcome and understand negative and distorted thinking. Most often used, CBT is a combination of behavioral and cognitive therapies.

Interpersonal therapy helps the person concentrate on building healthy relationships. Overall, talk therapy helps teach coping skills and new ways of interacting with others. Therapy is often used in conjunction with medication, but it can be effective without medication as well. The amount of talk therapy a person needs depends on the individual and the depression severity.

Antidepressants, anti-anxiety, and mood-stabilizing anticonvulsants are medications used to treat depression. Of those, antidepressants are the most common. There are several different antidepressant medications: selective serotonin reuptake inhibitors (SSRIs), tricyclics, and monoamine oxidase inhibitors (MAOIs). These medications must be taken regularly for three to four weeks before the full effect occurs, but some improvement can be seen within the first two weeks. Often people will stop taking their medication because they start to feel better, or because they do not feel the full effects immediately. However, it is important to continue taking the medication for approximately six months, or as prescribed, to prevent a reoccurrence of depression. Antidepressant medications are not habit-forming, but have to be closely monitored to ensure the correct dosage has been prescribed. Persons should be under the directions of a physician or psychiatrist when prescribed medication such as anti-anxiety drugs along with antidepressants. However, if taken alone, anti-anxiety drugs are not effective in treating a depressive disorder. The mood-stabilizing anticonvulsants are typically used to treat bipolar disorder and control associated mood swings. It is best, as with any medication, to work closely with your physician so the dosage can be carefully monitored for the best possible effectiveness.

Lifestyle changes, along with therapy and/or medication, can help improve depression symptoms. A healthy diet, yoga, meditation, and increased exercise have been shown to produce positive effects in those with depression. Exercise may increase energy and reduce stress to help fend off depression. Research indicates that even low-intensity exercise, such as walking, is beneficial to mental health. The increased levels of the hormone norepinephrine, found in the blood after exercise, helps the brain adjust to the stress that can lead to depression and anxiety. Through these lifestyle changes an individual can reverse the negative effects of depression.

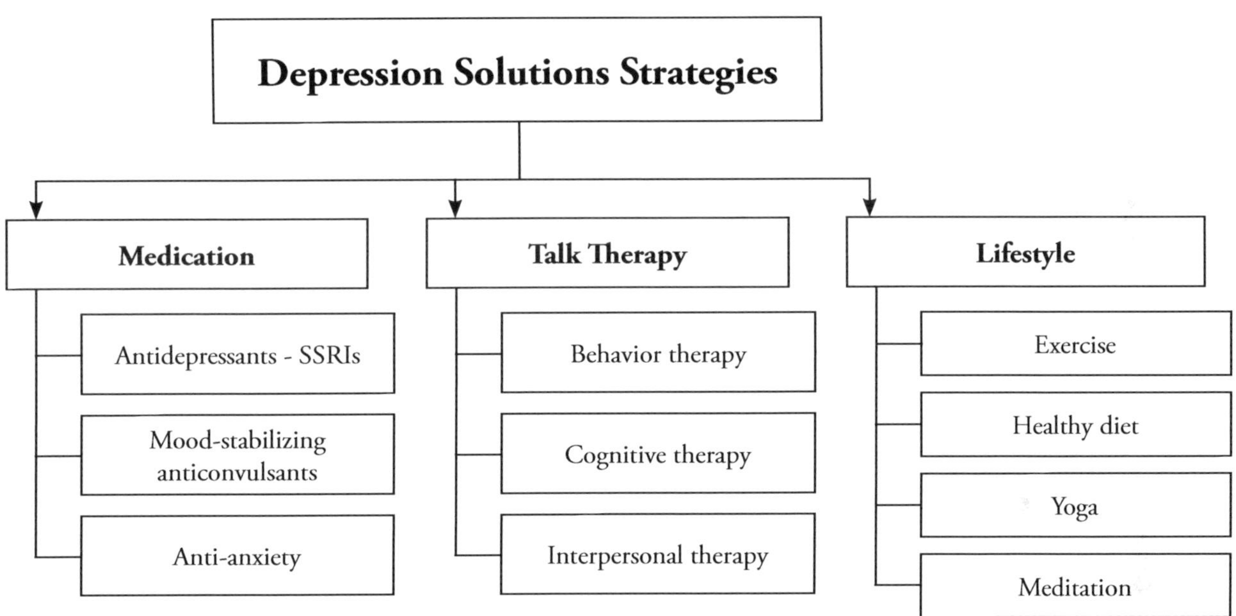

Depression is a serious disorder that can become life threatening if left untreated. While depression affects people differently, it is important to realize the negative effects and seek treatment as soon as possible. People with depression rarely just "snap out of it." With the proper treatment and support, negative feelings and thoughts can begin to fade over time. Depression is a treatable medical condition that should not be ignored. With the help of a health care professional, an appropriate and effective treatment can be developed. It is important to remember that depression does not have to affect your life, and there is help available.

Chapter 5 – Resiliency

Think about a traumatic event or challenge in your life that you were still able to overcome. This is commonly referred to as resiliency - a term that refers to an individuals' strength in the midst of change or stressful life events. It is the power a person has to spring back or recover from adversity. People who are resilient exhibit useful characteristics. These characteristics 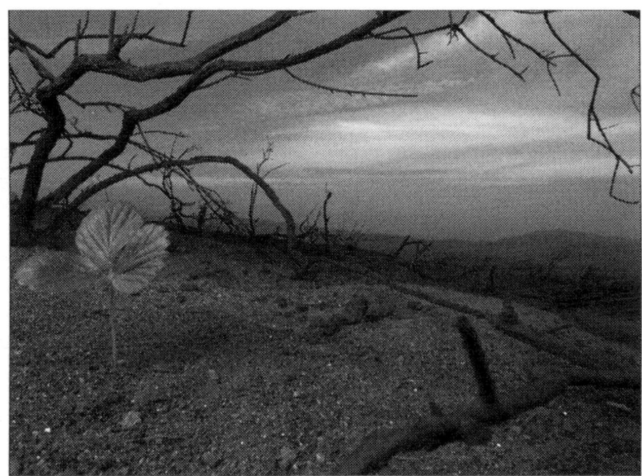 include, the ability to take responsibility, easily moving on with their life, and understanding situations in a positive manner. A resilient person has the ability to bounce back from a negative situation or challenge using their inner strength. Resiliency is helpful in stressful situations and can offer protection from depression, anxiety, and developing other disorders. The schematic below provides an overview of resiliency.

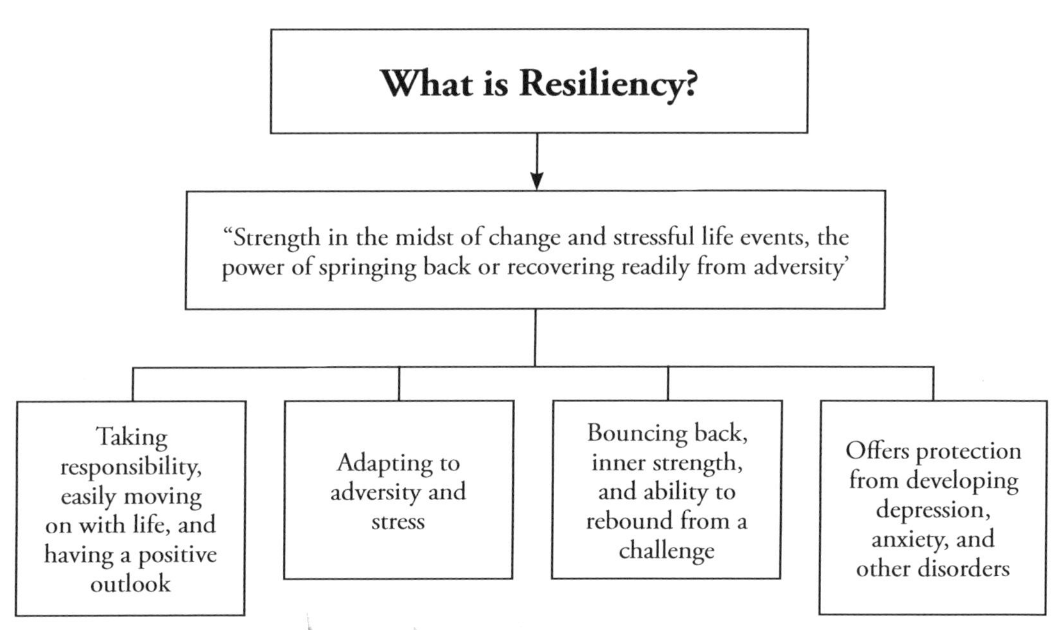

While resiliency is about adapting well to stress, adversity, trauma, or tragedy, it does not mean you have to ignore your feelings or that you cannot ask for support from others. Being able to reach out to others is important. There are nine separate elements of resilience (energy management, social support, attitude management, life goal planning, healthy diet, purposeful activity, stress relief, self-care, and creative fun) that contribute to the achievement of personal responsibility, empowerment, meaningful connections, and the ability to move on. These core elements are used to address a wide range of issues that contribute to an individual's overall health and well-being. They also attempt to find a balance between physical, psychological, intellectual, social, and spiritual facets of health. Each of these nine elements will be briefly explained. You will likely not use all of these. In fact, you may not agree that some of these work for you personally. However, these elements will provide you with useful options.

Energy management refers to your personal energy that contributes to your level of activity. It also contributes to your ability to take personal responsibility for life events. Energy management encompasses rest habits, physical activity patterns, use of "quiet" time, personal energy level awareness, and effort put into activities.

Creative fun is the ability to find humor and a creative outlook in life events. Whether you find a new way to re-interpret an event or find humor or lightness in your usual way, creative fun will help to conquer the dire-seriousness of many situations.

Attitude management involves the use of strategies to maintain a composed attitude. This element encompasses such strategies as anger management, intentional self-talk, use of coping strategies, and the awareness of your attitudes, emotions, and feelings.

Stress relief refers to the various relaxation strategies used to alleviate the effects of stress. The use of traditional management and prevention strategies related to stress will be helpful as well.

Life goal planning allows you to take time to focus on your life, what you want from it, and what direction you are moving towards. This element gives you the opportunity to determine your life purpose, major life goals, community contribution, career pursuits, and the balance between materialistic endeavors and spirituality.

A healthy diet as an element of resilience refers to the choice of more fruits and vegetables, lean meats, low fat dairy, and whole grains in place of excess oils, fats, and sweets. By choosing healthier food options you can enhance many aspects associated with your lifestyle including increased energy, disease prevention, increased or better sleep, and greater concentration throughout the day.

Purposeful activity focuses on making sure that work, recreation, and other activities are meaningful within your life. To maintain personal resilience it is important to have a clear purpose. A lack of purpose tends to negatively affect resiliency.

Social support involves the relationships in your life, currently or in the past, and the level of support you obtain from each of them. Relationships can include friends, co-workers, family, a significant other, or children. Social support encompasses the length of contact with an individual, the level of perceived support and intimacy, how often you have contact with a person, and the degree of openness you experience.

The self care element involves an individual's ability to recognize the signs and symptoms of lowered resilience and identify strategies that can be used to improve it.

Strategies for improving resilience include stretching, moderation, remaining flexible with life in general, taking rest breaks, quiet time, and change-of-focus exercises.

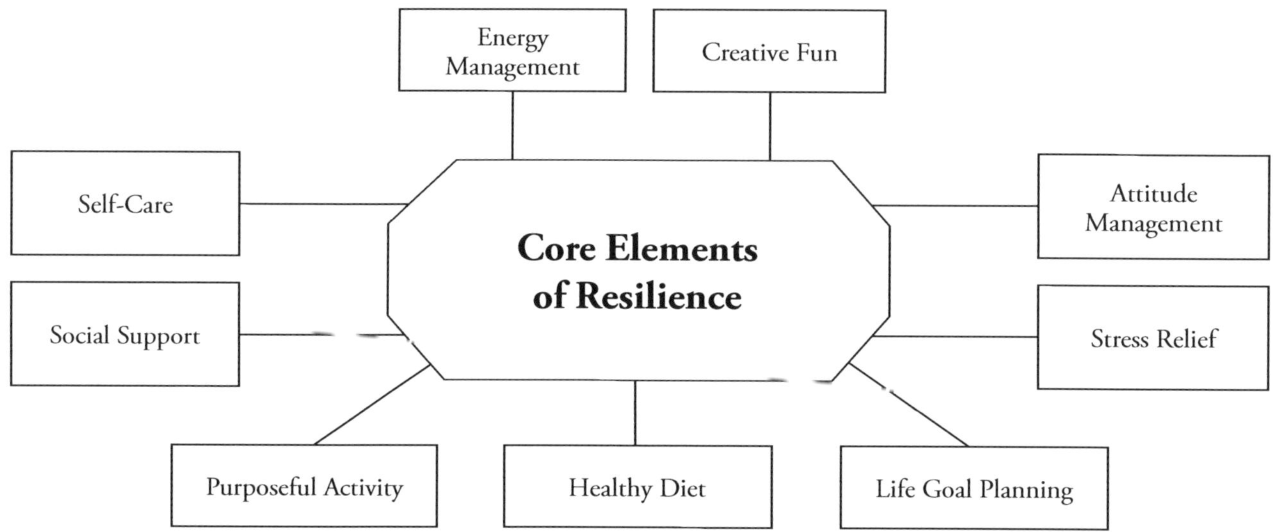

The strategies used in creating or improving resilience fall within these nine core elements. The strategies are a part of each of the core elements. These strategies help to nurture an individual's resilience and can be adapted to fit within your lifestyle or specific situation. These strategies include: making connections, accepting that change is a part of living, establishing realistic 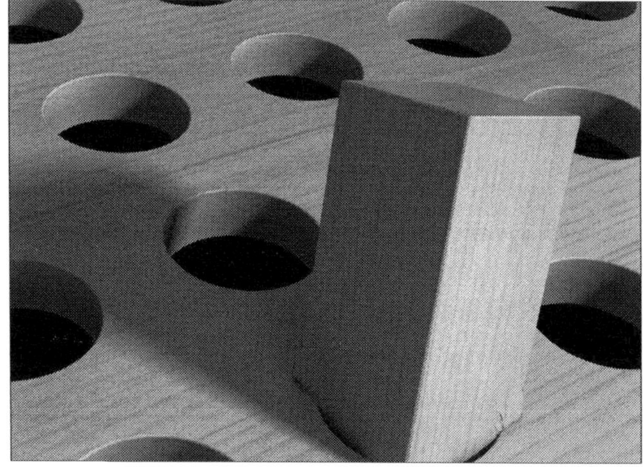 goals and moving toward them, taking action, rediscovering yourself, being positive about yourself, keeping it in perspective, being optimistic, taking care of yourself, learning from the past, and looking forward. Through the use of these strategies you can help to build a better sense of resiliency or improve a distressing situation.

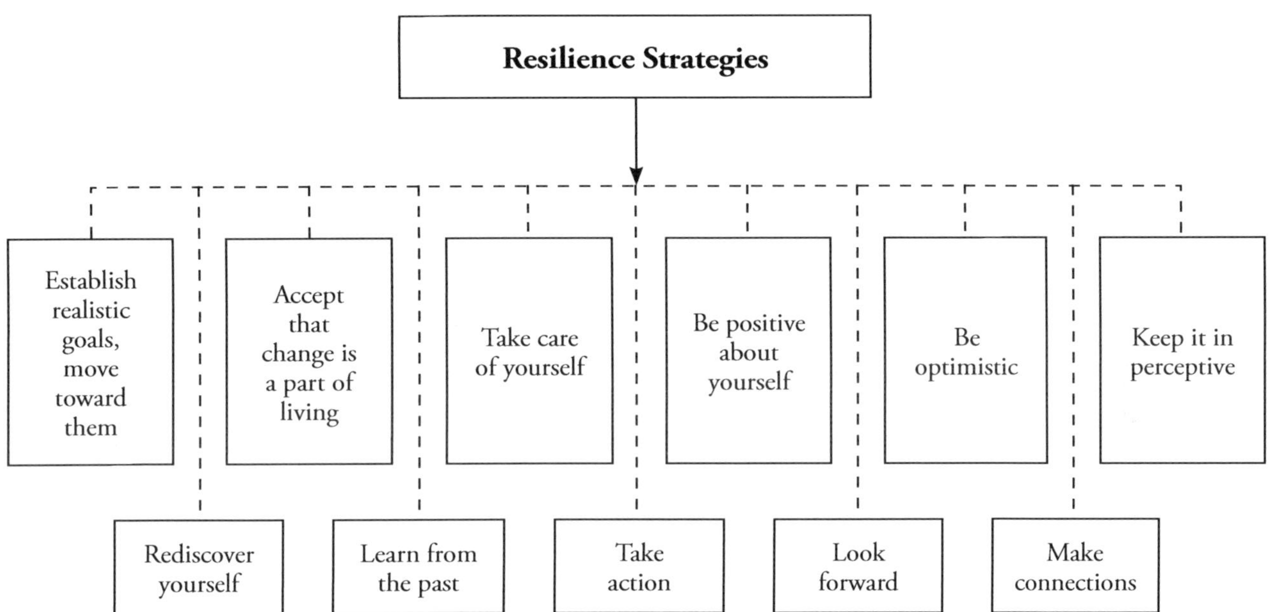

While resiliency is a helpful tool to navigate through stressful or traumatic situations, there are limitations. Resiliency is an individualized experience that cannot be forced upon anyone. You cannot make someone resilient; while you can provide the tools and resources necessary, they have to use them to experience the benefits. Resiliency is a great tool that can be used to find the lightness or humor in a situation, but remember it will not make your problems go away; it will only present an opportunity to make the situation better. Also, each strategy should be adapted to the person because resiliency is an individualized state.

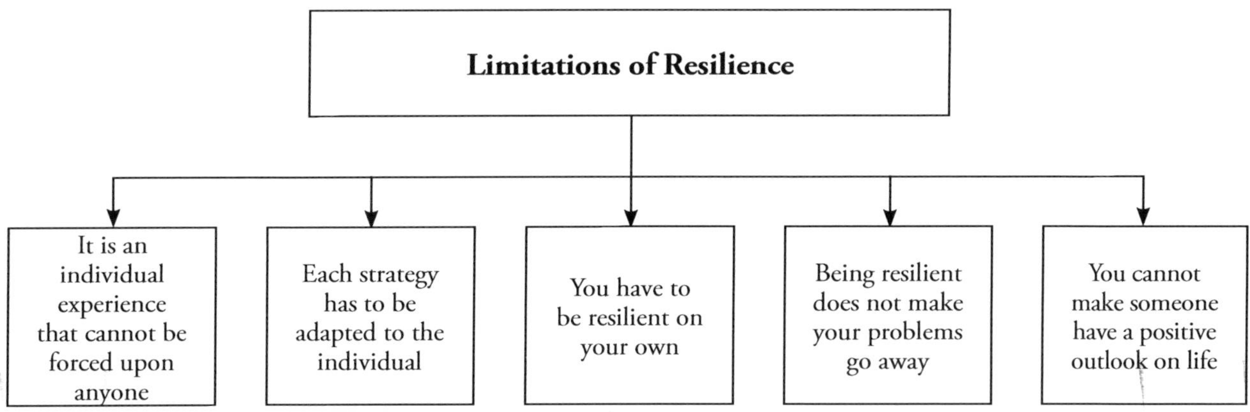

Resiliency can help you develop a reservoir of internal resources that you can draw from when you experience chronic stress, endure loss, or face other challenges. It can help you to thrive in the midst of chaos and difficult situations. Resilient individuals are described as individuals who have cultivated a sense of forgiveness, or those who possess a sense of emotional buoyancy. While resilient individuals still experience sadness, they choose to see situations in a positive manner and realize they cannot control all aspects of their life. It is important to remember how you think, how you act, and how you relate to others will have an impact on future situations.

Chapter 6 – Other Lifestyle Issues

Still having trouble sleeping? Have you ever thought your lifestyle may contribute? A good idea is to examine your lifestyle to determine if this might be a leading factor in causing you to have sleep troubles. Getting regular physical activity, eating a healthy diet, and managing chronic conditions will help combat the effects and symptoms of insomnia and other sleep disorders, and likely help you sleep better.

Regular physical activity has been shown to provide many benefits when dealing with fatigue and/or stress. Regular physical activity is defined as five or more days of moderate exercise a week for at least 30 minutes. The benefits associated with physical activity include having more energy, coping better with stress, increasing your resistance to stress, helping you to relax and feel less tense, improving productivity at work and therefore decreasing stress, and providing greater resistance to stress. It also helps you to counter anxiety and depression, fall asleep quickly and sleep well, build stamina for other activities, tone your muscles, and physical activity also helps your heart and lungs work more efficiently. Overall, physical activity helps you to feel better, look better, and function more efficiently. The schematic below outlines the benefits of physical activity.

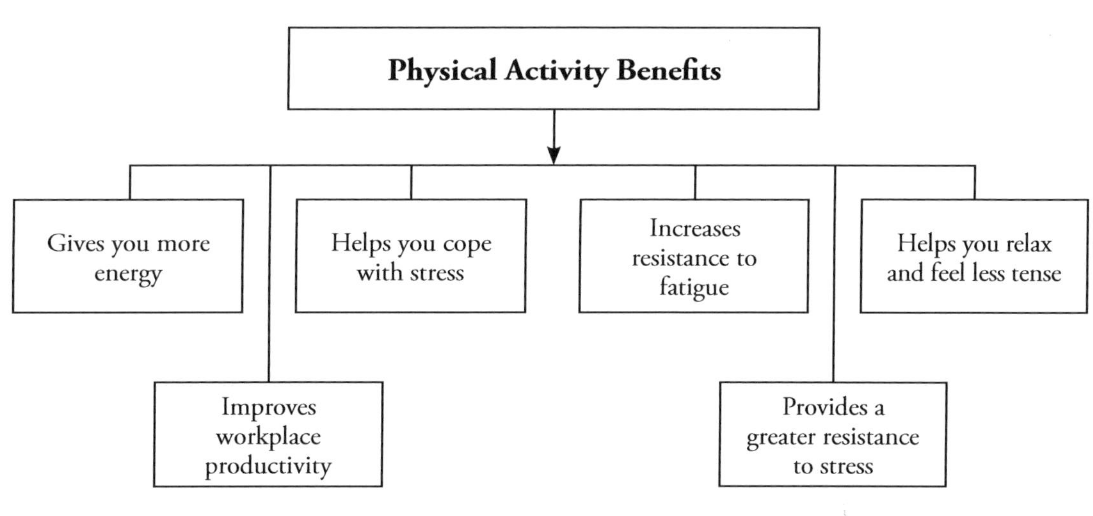

While regular physical activity is beneficial for improving sleep patterns, there are several considerations to take into account. The five rules to follow include talking to your doctor to identify what is safe for you, realizing your barriers, identifying your preferred mode(s) of activity, getting and staying motivated, and setting short- and long-term goals.

It is recommended to first consult your physician before beginning any physical activity. Talking with your healthcare provider will help you identify if your plans for physical activity are safe and right for you. It will also help you recognize any issues or health conditions that you may have that could harm or injure you if planning to increase your activity.

By identifying your barriers you will be able to confront and prevent them from getting in the way of you becoming more active. First, examine what barriers have prevented you from being active in the past, and then find ways to overcome each one. Common barriers include fear of injury, lack of time or facility, and fear of discomfort.

Choosing your mode of physical activity will determine your success. Start by identifying activities you enjoy. Do not choose activities you have never enjoyed in hopes that you will learn to. Chances are, you will not stay active if you do not enjoy the activity you select.

Motivation is key to your success. While it may be hard to find motivation at the beginning, it is helpful to keep in mind your goals and why you started becoming more physically active. Remember, the benefits you are gaining will likely far outweigh any negative aspects you may be experiencing. Enlisting social support is a great way to get and stay motivated.

Through the use of goal setting, you will be able to plan your physical activity. Start by identifying what you want to accomplish, and then break that goal down into small short-term goals. Write them down and post them in a place you will visit frequently. It may also be helpful to give your goals to a friend, family member, or co-worker to keep you on track. Lastly, make sure you reward yourself each time you accomplish one of your goals.

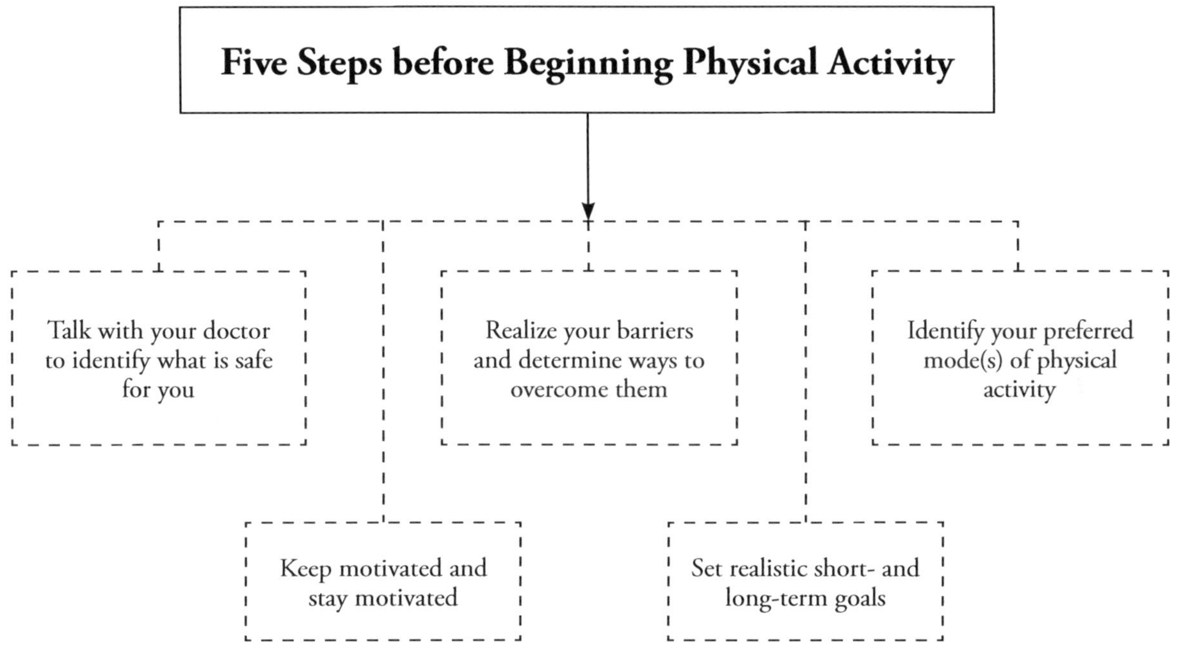

Starting a new physical activity regimen can seem difficult, and may be even a little scary. The following tips will help you slowly and safely increase the amount of physical activity in your life. These tips include wearing proper clothing, starting slow, getting enough rest, having the right equipment, asking for advice, educating yourself about physical activity, and finding new ways to be active.

Proper clothing is important when being active in various climates. Lightweight, breathable clothing is needed when active indoors or in high heat/humid conditions. Wearing several layers in colder temperatures is critical. Stay comfortable and avoid tight clothing that may cause irritation.

Starting slow and building up to your fitness goals is the best way to begin. Taking on too much, too fast greatly increases your chances for injury which could greatly hinder any progress you have made. It is better to be safe and work your way up than to injure yourself, or to push yourself too hard so that you give up early on. You will perform better at your chosen activity by starting slower.

Get plenty of rest and listen to your body. If you are experiencing pain or fatigue, this is your body trying to tell you something is wrong and you should stop immediately. While you may experience minor discomfort at the start of your activity regimen, you should never experience pain. Make sure you give injuries plenty of time to properly heal. Being active before you have had enough rest between sessions may lead to another injury.

Make sure you have the right equipment for your chosen activity. Safety equipment is a large part of the proper attire needed. Helmets, safety pads, and proper shoes are all part of being physically active, and serve an important purpose - injury prevention. Safety equipment is especially important when engaging in outside activities.

Consult a professional such as a personal trainer or other health professional for advice on use of equipment and proper techniques. It is important to get good advice, decrease your risk of injury, and improve your overall skills.

Continue to educate yourself. Even if you already participate in regular physical activity, it is always a good idea to learn more about exercising properly and new techniques. There are numerous websites, books, and magazine articles to help you.

Finding new ways to be active and different activities that interest you will help you stay motivated. Try various activities to decrease boredom and increase your skills. By continually finding new activity interests, you are more likely to maintain a regular physical activity program.

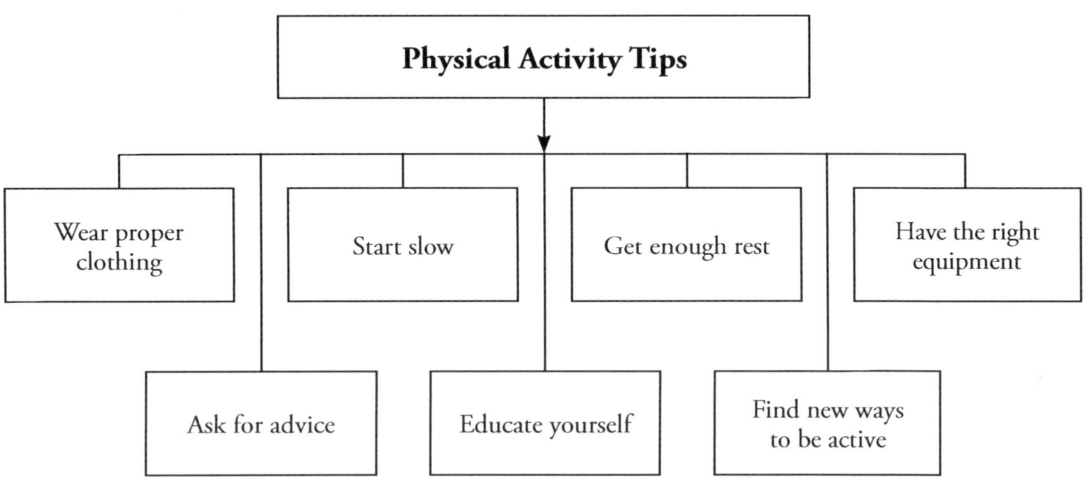

Proper nutrition is another lifestyle issue that may influence your daily sleep pattern. A healthy diet is crucial to maintaining a healthy weight, and preventing obesity and other conditions. Obesity can lead to type 2 diabetes, breathing problems such as sleep apnea, and psychological disorders such as depression, having an impact on your quality and quantity of sleep. The following nutrition tips will help you sleep better: incorporate more fruits and vegetables into your diet, eating healthier will make you feel and sleep better; avoid fad diets that will leave you feeling hungry and fatigued; do not go to sleep hungry, it can cause you to have trouble falling and staying asleep; and if hungry, eat a small, light carbohydrate meal before bed.

By incorporating more fruits and vegetables into your diet you will substitute your usual snacks and side items for lower calorie, high-fiber foods. Fruits and vegetables will also help you feel full longer, therefore cutting down on the number of times you eat and the quantity of food you consume. Eating healthy will make you feel less lethargic or fatigued throughout the day. By choosing healthy options instead of chips or a candy bar, you will be equipped with the energy you need.

Fad diets promise big results, but deliver very little. They do not work, and will leave you feeling hungry and fatigued because of unhealthy nutrient restrictions. The only way to lose or maintain weight is to eat healthy and be active within your daily routine.

Finally, choose a smaller meal for dinner rather than eating heavy. This will leave you comfortably full and not interrupt your sleep. However, if dinner doesn't hold you over, do not to go to bed hungry because that can cause difficulty for you to fall and stay asleep. Instead, eat a small snack consisting of a light carbohydrate before bed when hungry. Again, avoid overeating before bed, which can also interrupt your sleep. The light snack will satisfy your hunger, but not make you uncomfortably full.

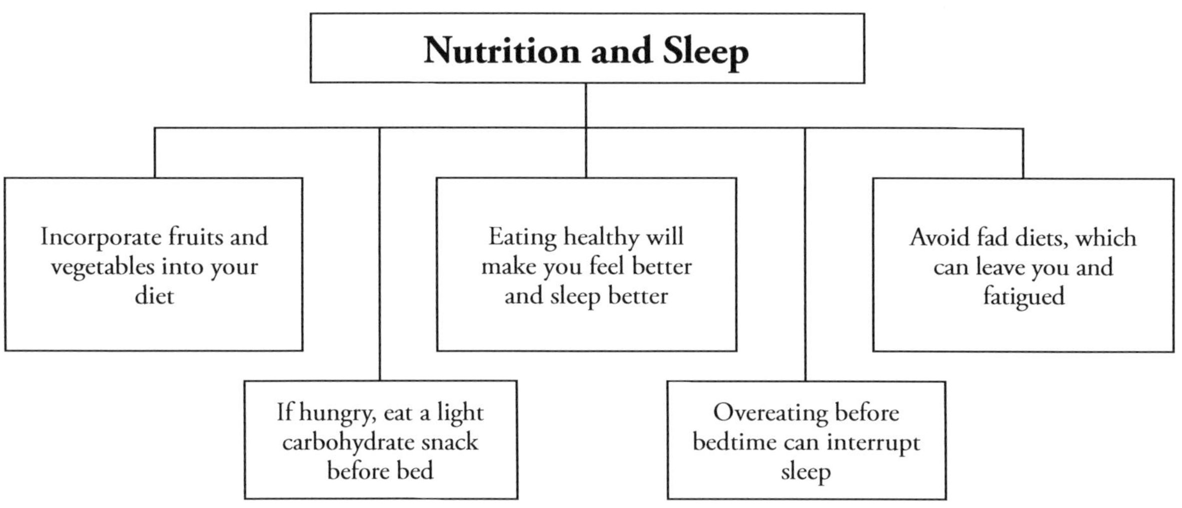

The final lifestyle issue we will discuss is management of chronic conditions, which can negatively affect your sleep. Chronic conditions include high cholesterol, hypertension, heart disease, diabetes, arthritis, cancers, and asthma. Each of these conditions has symptoms that affect the quality and quantity of your sleep. The schematic below provides an overview of the conditions that affect your sleep patterns.

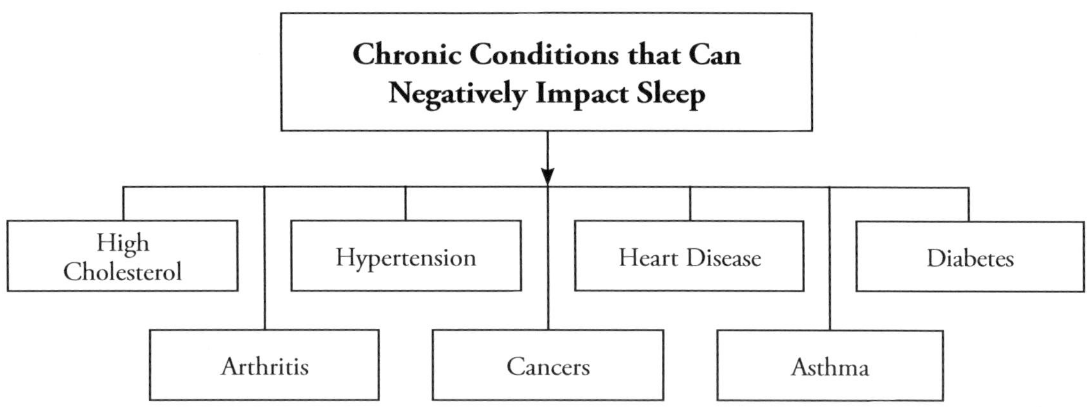

Fortunately, a healthy lifestyle and proper medical treatment may help to aid with managing or recovering from these chronic conditions. The healthy lifestyle components include proper nutrition, physical activity, plenty of sleep, managing stress, and social support. Through the practice of both physical activity and a proper diet, you will be able to prevent weight gain. Excess weight causes strain on your heart and increases your chances of heart disease, high blood pressure, and high cholesterol. Managing stress and getting plenty of sleep helps combat symptoms associated with these chronic conditions. Finally, social support will help you maintain a healthy lifestyle and give you a resource to talk with about your successes, barriers, and everyday struggles. Talking with someone can help alleviate excess stress and create accountability.

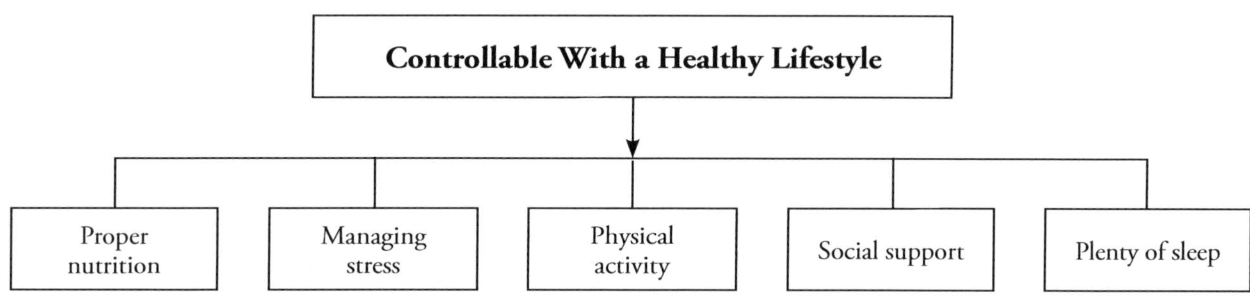

Physical activity, proper nutrition, and managing chronic conditions can play a critical role in your quality and quantity of sleep. By incorporating each of these lifestyle issues into your daily routine you will experience a better quality of life. All three lifestyle issues are interrelated and will lead you to better sleep.

Made in the USA
San Bernardino, CA
06 May 2020

71144855R00033